BLUEPRIN

Hematology and Oncology

Blueprints **for your pocket!**

In an effort to answer a need for high yield review books for the elective rotations, Blackwell Publishing now brings you Blueprints in pocket size.

These new Blueprints provide the essential content needed during the elective rotations. If you are looking for basic content to prepare for the USMLE Steps 2 and 3, or if you were unable to fit in the rotation, these new pocket-sized Blueprints are just what you need.

Each book will focus on the high yield essential content for the most commonly encountered problems of the specialty. Each book features these special appendices:

- Career and residency opportunities
- Commonly prescribed medications
- Self-test Q&A section

Ask for these at your medical bookstore or check them out online at www.blackwellmedstudent.com

Blueprints Dermatology
Blueprints Urology
Blueprints Pediatric Infectious Diseases
Blueprints Ophthalmology
Blueprints Plastic Surgery
Blueprints Orthopedics
Blueprints Hematology and Oncology
Blueprints Infectious Diseases

BLUEPRINTS
Hematology and Oncology

Casey O'Connell, MD
Fellow, Department of Hematology
Los Angeles County/University of Southern
California Medical Center
Los Angeles, California

Vanessa Lynn Dickey, MD
Attending Hematologist and Oncologist
Cancer Care Associates Medical Group, Inc.
Redondo Beach, California

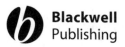
Blackwell
Publishing

Blackwell Publishing, Inc., 350 Main Street, Malden, Massachusetts 02148-5018, USA
Blackwell Publishing Ltd, 9600 Garsington Road, Oxford OX4 2DQ, UK
Blackwell Publishing Asia Pty Ltd, 550 Swanston Street, Carlton, Victoria 3053, Australia

05 06 07 08 5 4 3 2 1

ISBN-13: 978-1-4051-0449-4
ISBN-10: 1-4051-0449-X

Library of Congress Cataloging-in-Publication Data

O'Connell, Casey.
  Hematology and oncology/Casey O'Connell, Vanessa Lynn Dickey.
       p. ; cm.—(Blueprints)
  Includes index.
  ISBN-13: 978-1-4051-0449-4 (pbk.)
  ISBN-10: 1-4051-0449-X (pbk.)
  1. Hematology—Handbooks, manuals, etc. 2. Oncology—Handbooks, manuals, etc.
  [DNLM: 1. Hematology Diseases—Handbooks. 2. Lymphatic Diseases—Handbooks. 3. Neoplasms—Handbooks. WH 39 018h 2005]
  I. Dickey, Vanessa Lynn. II. Title. III. Series.
  RC633.026 2005
  616.99'418—dc22   2004026976

A catalogue record for this title is available from the British Library

Acquisitions: Beverly Copland
Development: Selene Steneck
Production: Debra Murphy
Illustrations: Electronic Illustrators Group
Cover design: Hannus Design Associates
Interior design: Mary McKeon
Typesetter: International Typesetting and Composition in Ft. Lauderdale, FL
Printed and bound by Capital City Press in Berlin, VT

For further information on Blackwell Publishing, visit our website:
www.blackwellmedstudent.com

Notice: The indications and dosages of all drugs in this book have been recommended in the medical literature and conform to the practices of the general community. The medications described do not necessarily have specific approval by the Food and Drug Administration for use in the diseases and dosages for which they are recommended. The package insert for each drug should be consulted for use and dosage as approved by the FDA. Because standards for usage change, it is advisable to keep abreast of revised recommendations, particularly those concerning new drugs.

Dedicated to patients everywhere suffering with cancer or a blood disorder.

A special thanks to Dr. Alexandra Levine and Dr. Donald Feinstein—the two best mentors in hematology and oncology. We are forever indebted to your generosity of spirit, compassion for the human race, and example as superb clinicians.

Contents

Reviewers

Mallar Bhattacharya, MD, MSc
PGY-1
The Johns Hopkins Hospital
Baltimore, Maryland

Celeste Chu Kuo, MD
Pediatrics Intern
St. Louis Children's Hospital
St. Louis, Missouri

Edmundo Justino, MD
PGY-1
Internal Medicine
Johns Hopkins Bayview Medical Center
Baltimore, Maryland

Jennifer Lai, MD
PGY-2
Santa Clara Valley Medical Center
San Jose, California

Eric Pacini, MD
Intern
University of Texas Southwestern Medical Center
Dallas, Texas

Devi SenGupta, MD, MPhil
PGY-1
The Johns Hopkins Hospital
Baltimore, Maryland

Sarah Kathleen Taylor, MD
1st year resident
Seattle Children's Hospital/University of Washington Medical Center
Seattle, Washington

Preface

Blueprints have become the standard for medical students to use during their clerkship rotations and sub-internships and as a review book before taking the USMLE Steps 2 and 3.

Blueprints initially were only available for the five main specialties: medicine, pediatrics, obstetrics, surgery, and psychiatry. Students found these books so valuable that they asked for Blueprints in other topics and so family medicine, emergency medicine, neurology, cardiology, and radiology were added.

In an effort to answer a need for high-yield review books for the elective rotations, Blackwell Publishing now brings you Blueprints in pocket size. These books are developed to provide students in the shorter, elective rotations, often taken in fourth year, with the same high-yield, essential contents of the larger Blueprints books. These new pocket-sized Blueprints will be invaluable for those students who need to know the essentials of a clinical area but were unable to take the rotation. Students in physician assistant, nurse practitioner, and osteopath programs will find these books meet their needs for the clinical specialties.

Feedback from student reviewers gives high praise for this addition to the Blueprints brand. Each of these new books was developed to be read in a short time and to address the basics needed during a particular clinical rotation. Please see the Series Page for a full list of the books in this series.

Abbreviations

ACA	Anticardiolipin antibodies
ACD	Anemia of chronic disease
ACS	Acute chest syndrome
ACTH	Adrenocorticotropic hormone
ADH	Antidiuretic hormone
AFP	α-Fetoprotein
AJCC	American Joint Committee on Cancer
ALA	Aminolevulinic acid
ALL	Acute lymphocytic leukemia
AML	Acute myeloid leukemia
AMM	Agnogenic myeloid metaplasia
ANC	Absolute neutrophil count
APC	Activated C protein
APC	Adenomatous polyposis coli
APL	Acute promyelocytic leukemia
aPTT	Activated partial thromboplastin time
ARDS	Acute respiratory distress syndrome
ASCUS	Atypical squamous cells of unknown significance
AT	Antithrombin
ATG	Antithymocyte globulin
ATRA	All-trans retinoic acid
BPH	Benign prostatic hyperplasia
Ca	Calcium
CABG	Coronary artery bypass graft
CaEDTA	Chelation
CBC	Complete blood (cell) count
CEA	Carcinoembryonic antigen
CEP	Congenital erythropoietic porphyria
CHF	Congestive heart failure
CHOP	Cytoxan, adriamycin, vincristine, prednisone
CIN	Cervical intraepithelial neoplasia
CIS	Carcinoma *in situ*
CLL	Chronic lymphocytic leukemia
CMD	Chronic myeloproliferative disorders
CML	Chronic myeloid leukemia
CMML	Chronic myelomonocytic leukemia
CMV	Cytomegalovirus
CNS	Central nervous system
CRP	C-reactive protein

CXR	Chest x-ray
CS	Congenital spherocytosis
CT	Computed tomography
CVP	Cytoxan, vincristine, prednisone
DAT	Direct Coombs test
DCIS	Ductal carcinoma *in situ*
DDAVP	Desmopressin
DES	Diethylstilbestrol
DIC	Disseminated intravascular coagulation
DLCO	Diffusing capacity for carbon monoxide
DRE	Digital rectal examination
DVT	Deep venous thrombosis
EBT	Exchange blood transfusion
EBV	Epstein-Barr virus
EDTA	Edetate calcium disodium
EGF	Epidermal growth factor
ELISA	Enzyme-linked immunosorbent assay
EPO	Erythropoietin
ERCP	Endoscopic retrograde cholangiopancreatography
ESR	Erythrocyte sedimentation rate
ET	Essential thrombocythemia
FAMM	Familial atypical mole-melanoma
FAP	Familial adenomatous polyposis
FCL	Follicular lymphoma
FFP	Fresh frozen plasma
FIGO	International Federation of Gynecology and Obstetrics
FISH	Fluorescence *in situ* hybridization
FNA	Fine needle aspiration
G6PD	Glucose-6-phosphate dehydrogenase
GFR	Glomerular filtration rate
GI	Gastrointestinal
GU	Genitourinary
GVHD	Graft-versus-host disease
H&P	History and physical
Hb	Hemoglobin
HBV	Hepatitis B virus
HCC	Hepatocellular carcinoma
hCG	Human chorionic gonadotropin
HCL	Hairy cell leukemia
Hct	Hematocrit
HD	Hodgkin disease
HDL	High-density lipoprotein
HELLP	Hemolysis, elevated liver enzymes, low platelets
HGSIL	High-grade squamous intraepithelial lesion
HHM	Humoral hypercalcemia of malignancy
HHV-8	Human herpesvirus-8
HIT	Heparin-induced thrombocytopenia
HIV	Human immunodeficiency virus

HLA	Human leukocyte antigen
HNPCC	Hereditary nonpolyposis colorectal cancer
HPA-1a	Human platelet antigen-1a
HPV	Human papillomavirus
HRPC	Hormone-refractory prostate cancer
HTLV-1	Human T-cell leukemia virus-1
HUS	Hemolytic uremic syndrome
IFN	Interferon
Ig	Immunoglobulin
IgA	Immunoglobulin A
IgD	Immunoglobulin D
IgG	Immunoglobulin G
IgM	Immunoglobulin M
INR	International normalized ratio
ITD	Inherited thrombotic disorder
ITP	Idiopathic thrombocytopenic purpura
IV	Intravenous
IVC	Inferior vena cava
IVIg	Intravenous immunoglobulin
IVP	Intravenous pyelogram
LA	Lupus anticoagulant
LCIS	Lobular carcinoma *in situ*
LD	Lymphocyte depleted
LDH	Lactate dehydrogenase
LDL	Low-density lipoprotein
LDT	Lymphocyte doubling time
LEEP	Loop electrosurgical excision procedure
LFT	Liver function test
LGSIL	Low-grade squamous intraepithelial lesion
LHRH	Luteinizing hormone–releasing hormone
LMWH	Low-molecular-weight heparin
LP	Lymphocyte predominant
LPL	Lymphoplasmacytic lymphoma
MAHA	Microangiopathic hemolytic anemia
MALT	Mucosal-associated lymphoid tissue
MC	Mixed cellularity
MCL	Mantle cell lymphoma
MCV	Mean corpuscular volume
MDS	Myelodysplastic syndrome
MGUS	Monoclonal gammopathy of undetermined significance
MI	Myocardial infarction
MMA	Methylmalonic acid
MOA	Mechanism of action
MPV	Mean platelet volume
MRI	Magnetic resonance imaging
MUD	Matched unrelated donor
M-VAC	Methotrexate, vinblastine, adriamycin, cisplatin
MZL	Marginal zone lymphoma

NHL	Non-Hodgkin lymphoma
NS	Nodular sclerosis
NSAID	Nonsteroidal antiinflammatory drug
PA	Pernicious anemia
PAI-1	Plasminogen activator inhibitor-1
PCOS	Polycystic ovarian syndrome
PCR	Polymerase chain reaction
PE	Pulmonary embolism
PK	Pyruvate kinase
PI	Phospholipid
PML	Promyelocytic leukemia
PMN	Polymorphonuclear
PNH	Paroxysmal nocturnal hemoglobinuria
PO	By mouth
POMC	Proopiomelanocortin
PRCA	Pure red cell aplasia
PSA	Prostate-specific antigen
PT	Prothrombin time
PTHrp	Parathyroid hormone–related peptide
PV	Polycythemia vera
RA	Refractory anemia
RAR-α	Retinoic acid receptor-α
RBC	Red blood cell
RDW	Red cell distribution
RI	Reticulocyte index
RPLND	Retroperitoneal lymph node dissection
RT	Reverse transcriptase
S.E.	Side effects
SIADH	Syndrome of inappropriate secretion of antidiuretic hormone
SLE	Systemic lupus erythematosus
SLNB	Sentinel lymph node biopsy
SPEP	Serum protein electrophoresis
SVC	Superior vena cava
TF	Tissue factor
TIBC	Total iron binding capacity
TID	Twice daily
TNF	Tumor necrosis factor
TNM	Tumor, node, metastasis
TPA	Tissue plasminogen activator
TSH	Thyroid-stimulating hormone
TTE	Transthoracic echocardiogram
TTP	Thrombotic thrombocytopenic purpura
TUR	Transurethral resection
US	Ultrasound
VAD	Vincristine, adriamycin, Decadron
VEGF	Vascular epidermal growth factor

vWf	von Willebrand factor
WBC	White blood cell
WHO	World Health Organization
WT	Wild type
ZAP	Zeta-associated protein

Overview

Oncogenesis

Malignancy is thought to arise from the interaction of genetic changes and environmental factors. Genetic changes can be inherited from parents through the germline, meaning that every cell in the body will carry the mutant gene. For example, the inheritance of germline mutations in the BRCA1 or BRCA2 gene confers a significantly elevated risk of breast cancer; these mutations can be detected in the patient's normal cells before the onset of malignancy.

Genetic changes deemed **somatic mutations** occur in a given cell or tissue sporadically or as a result of external influences; they are not inherited. For example, when somatic mutations arise in the tumor suppressor gene known as p53, various cancers may ensue. One such mutation can be induced by smoking.

In either case, the presence of the genetic mutation alone is usually not enough to result in cancer. Other contextual factors, either genetic or environmental, are usually involved. For example, in the inherited genetic disorder **xeroderma pigmentosum**, a defective genetic repair gene leads to malignancy only after a certain level of ultraviolet (UV) exposure induces irreparable DNA mismatching in skin cells.

Important Terms

A **proto-oncogene** is a normal gene that has a high probability of leading to malignancy if it becomes mutated. Proto-oncogenes can become oncogenes through various mechanisms: loss of regulatory control via mutations in other genes, retroviral or other exogenous alteration of DNA leading to altered protein products, or accumulation of mutations resulting from absent DNA repair mechanisms.

An **oncogene** is a gene that is directly responsible for neoplastic tissue growth and can be classified as promotor oncogenes or tumor suppressor oncogenes. **Promoter oncogenes** overstimulate cell growth, development, and proliferation in cancer; e.g., the gene for the cell signaling enzyme tyrosine kinase, "abl," becomes an oncogene when translocated next to "bcr" in chronic myeloid leukemia. **Tumor suppressor oncogenes** become incapable of their usual tasks such as DNA repair, suppression of DNA promoter regions, and induction of apoptosis. Mutations in the p53 tumor suppressor gene are among the most common and have been implicated in various human cancers.

Microsatellite instability refers to inefficient repair of mismatched DNA pairs in short, apparently nonsense repeat sequences of DNA. Unfortunately, these sequences can occur in proto-oncogenes such as those that produce apoptosis and cell-cycle regulators. **MSH2** and **MLH1** are genes involved in mismatch repair that when mutated result in microsatellite instability; germline mutations in these genes have been implicated in the hereditary nonpolyposis colorectal cancer syndrome.

Role of Infections In Oncogenesis

Various infectious agents have been implicated in oncogenesis:
- Viruses can act by incorporating their own genetic material into the host's cellular genome.
- Viruses and bacteria can both act by chronically irritating tissue, causing cellular proliferation and increasing the chance of somatic mutations.

Some of the common malignancies associated with infections are listed in Table 1-1.

■ TABLE 1-1 Malignancies Associated with Infectious Agents

Malignancy	Associated Infectious Agent
Cervical cancer	Human papillomavirus
Gastric cancer	*Helicobacter pylori*
Hepatocellular carcinoma	Hepatitis B and hepatitis C viruses
Kaposi sarcoma	HHV-8
Primary effusion lymphoma	HHV-8
Splenic lymphoma	Hepatitis C virus
Nasopharyngeal carcinoma	EBV
Burkitt lymphoma	EBV
Adult T-cell leukemia/lymphoma	Human T-cell leukemia virus-1
Various lymphomas	HIV

EBV, Epstein-Barr virus; HHV-8, human herpesvirus-8; HIV, human immunodeficiency virus.

Benign Hematology

Peripheral Blood Basics

A generous amount of information can be obtained from reviewing a peripheral smear. This is the most important part of a hematologist's arsenal. A picture is worth a thousand words. Reliance on automated blood cell analysis is fraught with problems. There is no substitution for viewing a peripheral smear. Systematic scanning of blood smears helps the clinician avoid missing abnormal cells.

First, each smear should be examined with a 10× objective to assess the best area of the slide (i.e., where the red blood cells [RBCs] are evenly spread and just barely touching each other). If the smear is spread too thick with cells, the RBCs will be one on top of another, appearing superimposed. This can mimic "rouleaux," RBCs simulating a stack of coins.

Second, one should change to a 40× objective and assess for normal RBC morphology, which includes normal biconcave shape and RBCs of mostly all the same size.

RBCs should appear reddish-orange and have normal area of central pallor spanning half the cell diameter. RBCs average 7 μm in diameter. Comparing a cell of interest to an adjacent RBC can be helpful.

Neutrophils (or polymorphonuclear [PMN] cells) can be visualized at the 40× objective as two to five segmented lobes of the nucleus with purplish granules. PMN cells are bigger than an RBC, approximately 10 to 15 μm. A band form is an earlier PMN cell with a nucleus that never constricts to the point of a filament. Hypersegmented PMN cells are defined as greater than or equal to six nuclear segments. Most PMNs have four or more lobes. One should also see approximately six to seven platelets, fragments of round to oval blue-gray cells with red granules. Platelets are 2 μm. Platelets larger than 7 μm (the size of a normal RBC) are called giant platelets.

Lymphocytes have thin, pale blue cytoplasm and a dense, dark-staining nucleus approximately the same size as an RBC. There are usually no granules in lymphocytes. Occasionally lymphocytes can have more abundant cytoplasm and can reach sizes larger than an RBC, up to 15 μm.

Monocytes are much bigger than an RBC, even bigger than a neutrophil. The average size is 12 to 20 μm. The nucleus is usually indented, with sparse pick granules and gray-blue vacuoles.

Eosinophils are distinct by their numerous large red granules and bi-lobed nuclei. The usual size for an eosinophil is 10 to 15 μm.

Basophils are filled with large dark purplish to blue granules, usually with a bi-lobed nucleus. The average size of a basophil is 10 to 15 μm.

The third step is to advance to 50× and 100× using oil immersion for better viewing of granules and other features of the cells.

Peripheral Smears

Proficiency at evaluating blood smears involves practice and patience. Several peripheral smears are displayed in Plates 1 through 13 (see the color insert) for your inspection. A list of peripheral smears and dialogue follow. Many board examinations expect proficiency in the basic cells mentioned earlier. Attempt to identify the cells before reading the explanation.

Plate 1: The smear displays a band neutrophil on the left (note the indentation in the nucleus) and a normal neutrophil on the right. Also, several platelets with normal granularity and size are displayed. Red blood cell morphology is normal in this smear.

Plate 2: A neutrophil is displayed with a normal-appearing lymphocyte. Note the pale thin cytoplasm of the lymphocyte and the corresponding size to a red blood cell, almost the same size. Four to five platelets are also present.

Plate 3: A typical monocyte is displayed, which is clearly larger than a red blood cell with characteristic vacuoles.

Plate 4: A basophil with dark granules almost obscuring the nucleus.

Plate 5: Three prominent eosinophils are present with red granules.

Plate 6: This smear demonstrates a Pelger-Huet neutrophil on the left. This cell is a neutrophil with two round lobes connected by a single thin filament. The nuclear chromatin is denser and darker than a normal polymorphonuclear (PMN) cell. This cell is commonly seen in myelodysplasia and heritable disorders. Note the normal PMN band and lymphocyte.

Plate 7: Rouleaux (i.e., stack of coins) is displayed on this smear. This can be an artifact found in the thick areas of a smear. Four or more red blood cells (RBCs) stacked in a linear arrangement defines rouleaux. Normally, RBCs repel each other because of the negative charge on their surface. Increased amounts of fibrinogen or globulins (as in multiple myeloma) attach to the negatively charged RBCs, causing a net positive charge, and the cells stick together.

Plate 8: Toxic granulation of polymorphonuclear (PMN) cells is manifest by large dark blue granules with vacuoles. Vacuoles are the sites of digestion of phagocytized material. Toxic granulation is commonly seen in infections, trauma, burns, and after growth factors.

Plate 9: This slide displays the crescentic cells of a patient with sickle cell. Repeated sickling leads to irreversibly sickled cells. Also, note the target cells with a dense center appearing targetoid, or as a bull's eye. Increased surface membrane-volume ratio results in a central darker region within the normal area of pallor. Targets can be seen in many diseases, including sickle cell, liver disease, and thalassemia. Targets are also referred to as codocytes.

Plate 10: This slide demonstrates a classic smear for thrombotic thrombocytopenic purpura (TTP). Numerous fragmented cells, schistocytes, helmet cells, and keratocytes are displayed. All have irregular cell shape and lack central pallor. These cells are created during fragmentation as the cell traverses the bloodstream. The cells shear off in the microcirculation because of fibrin or occlusion. This slide could be seen in TTP, microangiopathic anemia, disseminated intravascular coagulation, uremia, malignant hypertension, valve hemolysis, and hemolytic uremic syndrome.

Plate 11: Acute leukemia with blasts on slide. First, note the large size of the blasts in relationship to the red blood cell, as well as the faint nucleoli present in each of these cells. This slide demonstrates acute leukemia; the subtype is not evident from this slide. Many times one cannot differentiate an acute myeloid leukemia blast from an acute lymphocytic leukemia blast. All the clinician can evaluate from this slide is leukemic blasts.

Plate 12: Multiple lymphocytes suggests chronic lymphocytic leukemia.

Plate 13: Hemolytic anemia: Spherocytes that are round and thicker than normal without central pallor are displayed. Spherocytes can be seen in hereditary spherocytosis and autoimmune hemolytic anemia. Also, note the polychromatophilic (blueish) red blood cell (RBC), indicative of early RBC turnover. A blueish cell reveals a small amount of RNA, a cell that left the bone marrow slightly early. On supravital staining, this cell would be considered a reticulocyte.

Clotting Cascade

- The clotting cascade (Figures 3-1 and 3-2) is a series of subsequent amplification steps leading to the formation of a fibrin clot.
- Each reaction requires four components: enzyme, cofactor, calcium (Ca), and phospholipid (Pl) surface.
- Coagulation proteins are serine protease enzymes or cofactors.
- Enzymes: Factor IIa, VIIa, IXa, Xa, tissue plasminogen activator (TPA), plasmin, protein C.
- Cofactors: tissue factor (TF), factor V, factor VIII, protein S.
- Others: Fibrinogen, factor XIII, antiplasmin, antithrombin, plasminogen activator inhibitor-1 (PAI-1).

Extrinsic Pathway

- TF and factor VIIa initiate the extrinsic pathway.
- TF is derived from brain, different animal sources, or human brain extract.
- It is called the extrinsic pathway because the TF is extrinsic, or added to, the pathway.
- In the body, TF is present on subendothelial surfaces and monocytes. It is released as a result of injury to vessels or endotoxin exposure on monocytes.
- The extrinsic pathway is tested by the prothrombin time (PT).
- Coumadin affects this pathway namely by inhibiting the vitamin K–dependent factors: II, VII, IX, and X, and protein C and S.
- An isolated prolonged PT implies a factor VII deficiency, vitamin K deficiency, liver disease, or an acquired inhibitor to factor VII.

■ Intrinsic Pathway

- Nothing is added to this pathway; thus it is named the intrinsic pathway.
- When the blood makes contact with glass (as in a test tube), factor XII activates factor XI.
- The intrinsic pathway is tested by the activated partial thromboplastin time (aPTT).

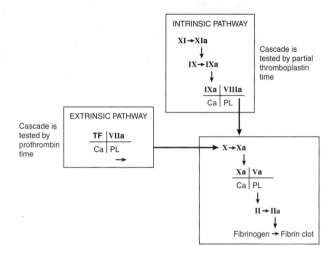

Figure 3-1 • Traditional clotting cascade

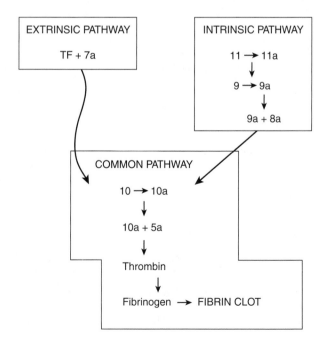

Figure 3-2 • Clotting cascade.

- Heparin affects this pathway by enhancing the anticoagulant property of antithrombin III.
- Isolated prolongation of the aPTT can mean many different diagnoses: heparin use, hemophilia, lupus anticoagulant, or factor inhibitors.
- Isolated shortening of aPTT indicates an elevated factor VIII.

■ Common Pathway

- Factors X and V are activated by the intrinsic and extrinsic pathways. This leads to thrombin formation and the fibrin clot.
- Thrombin is the most potent enzyme in the pathway and has many functions.
- Thrombin cleaves fibrinogen into fibrin, activates factor V and VIII, activates platelets, activates protein C, activates factor XIII, activates fibrinolysis, and activates factor XI, which initiates the intrinsic pathway and provides a positive feedback loop.

■ Fibrin Formation (Figure 3-3)

- The goal of the clotting cascade is to form a fibrin clot and prevent bleeding.
- Thrombin is key in converting fibrinogen to fibrin. Fibrin monomer is then converted to a more solid fibrin polymer by factor XIII.

■ Anticoagulants (Figure 3-4)

- Various proteins inactivate clotting factors.
- TF pathway inhibitor: Inhibits factor VII by binding to factors X and VIIa.
- Protein C: Binds factors Va and VIIIa, with cofactor protein S, inactivates factor V and factor VIII. Protein C and S are both

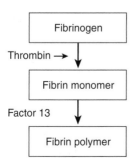

Figure 3-3 • Formation of fibrin clot

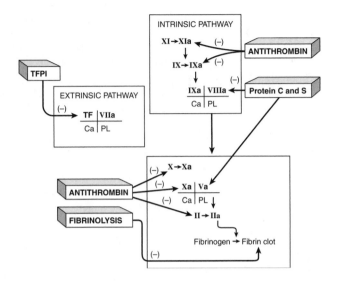

Figure 3-4 • Anticoagulants

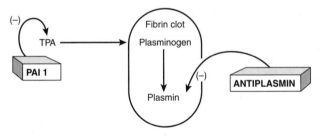

Figure 3-5 • Fibrinolytic pathway

vitamin K factors. Protein S circulates in a free form and a bound form. The free form binds and serves as the cofactor for protein C.

- Antithrombin: Binds and inactivates all the factors of the clotting cascade. Heparin accelerates this process.

■ **Fibrinolysis** (Figure 3-5)

- The fibrinolytic pathway serves to break down fibrin clots once they are formed. The enzymes work directly on the fibrin clot and all the reactions take place directly on fibrin.

- Plasminogen: Inactive precursor of plasmin. It is converted to plasmin by TPA.
  - TPA: Released by endothelial cells and converts plasminogen to plasmin.
  - Plasmin: Cleaves bonds in fibrin and fibrinogen, and breaks down the fibrin clot.
  - PAI-1: Produced by the liver and endothelial cells, and activated by endotoxin or thrombin. It binds and inactivates TPA.
  - Antiplasmin: Binds and inactivates plasmin; made by the liver. This is depleted in disseminated intravascular coagulation and liver disease and contributes to a bleeding diathesis.

4

Overview of Anemia

■ Definitions

- **Acanthocytes**: Red blood cells (RBCs) with thorny projections around their surface.
- **Anisocytosis**: Variation in the size of RBCs on a peripheral smear.
- **Hemoglobin (Hb)**: A tetramer of four globin chains whose function is to use iron to carry oxygen to human tissue.
  - 96% of adult Hb is Hb A, which consists of two α- and two β-globin chains.
  - 3% of adult Hb is Hb A_2 (two α- and two δ-globin chains).
  - 1% is fetal hemoglobin (Hb F) (two α- and two γ-globin chains).
- **Hematocrit (Hct)**: The percentage of whole blood volume that contains RBCs.
- **Mean corpuscular volume (MCV)**: The average volume of an RBC that corresponds to a diameter of about 7 μm on the peripheral smear.
- **RBC distribution width (RDW)**: A measure of the degree of difference in size between RBCs.
- **Reticulocytosis**: A bone marrow response to decreased Hb in which there is early release of immature RBCs.
  - On the peripheral smear, reticulocytes are larger and more basophilic (bluer) than normal RBCs.
- **Schistocytes**: Irregular, fragmented RBCs result from mechanical destruction in the peripheral blood, as seen in microangiopathic hemolytic anemias (fibrin strands slice the RBCs as they pass through the microcirculation) and in patients with artificial heart valves.
- **Spherocytes**: Small, smooth, round RBCs seen in congenital spherocytosis and autoimmune hemolytic anemia (splenic removal of immunoglobulins releases smaller more compact RBCs).
- **Target cell**: Erythrocyte with a central red "bull's eye" that is surrounded by central pallor and then an outer red ring, as seen in the hemoglobinopathies.
- **Hypochromia**: When the central pallor of erythrocytes exceeds one third of the cell's diameter, as seen in iron deficiency anemia

Plates

Please see chapter two for descriptions of these peripheral smears.

(All plates provided courtesy of Eric F. Glassy, M.D., Affiliated Pathologists Medical Group - Torrance, CA)

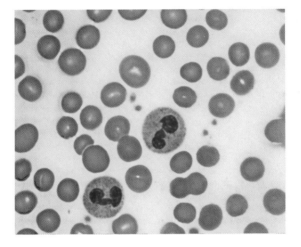

Plate 1 •

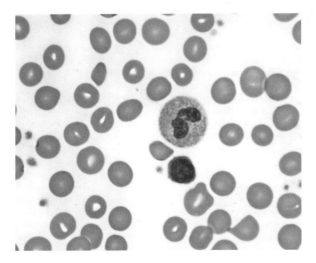

Plate 2 •

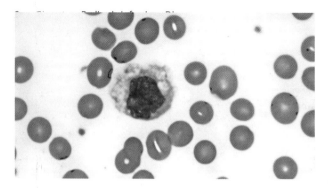

Plate 3 •

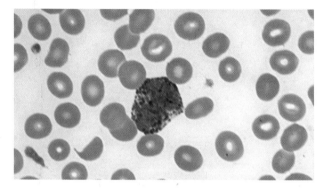

Plate 4 •

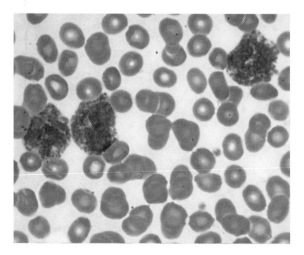

Plate 5 •

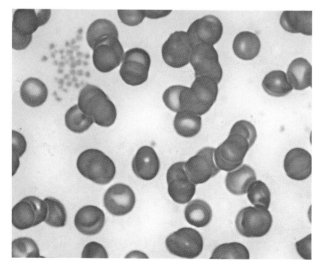

Plate 6 •

Plate 7 •

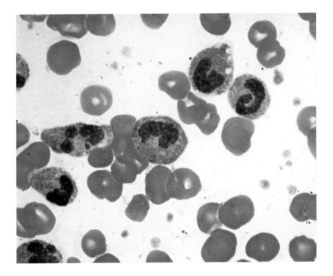

Plate 8 •

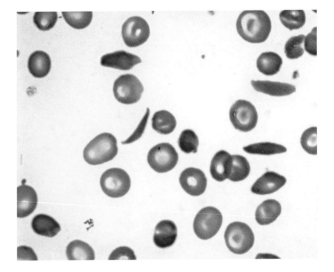

Plate 9 •

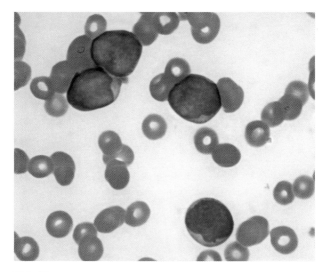

Plate 10 •

Plate 11 •

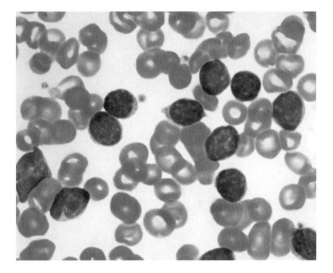

Plate 12 •

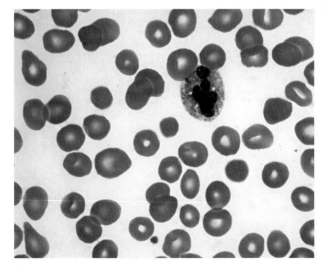

Plate 13 •

(the less Hb in the cell, the less stain that is taken up by the cell).

■ Laboratory Values and Interpretation

- **Hb**: The normal range in men is 13.5 to 17.0 g/dL; for women, 12 to 15 g/dL.
  - These numbers are based on 95% confidence intervals in an average population; however, the mean may vary based on age, race/ethnicity, geography, and other factors.
  - Anemia in the elderly is abnormal and should not be overlooked as "aging."
  - Testosterone increases the mean Hb values in men; before puberty, the gender disparity is not apparent.
  - The value is a concentration (grams per deciliter of whole blood), so it is affected by the plasma volume (see explanation in the next bulleted item).
- **Hct**: The normal range in men is 39% to 49%; for women, 33% to 43%.
  - This reflects the number of RBCs *relative to* the volume of whole blood, so the number can be falsely high immediately after massive blood loss. As fluid from the interstitium leaks into the blood vessels after a bleed, a process that can take up to 48 to 72 hours, the Hb and Hct become a more accurate reflection of the amount of blood lost.
- **MCV**: The normal range is 80 to 100 fL.
- **RDW**: Normal ranges are generated by the individual laboratory (usually around 12)
- **Reticulocyte count**: In a nonanemic patient, the bone marrow replaces about 1% of the RBC population daily.
  - The reticulocyte lasts about 3 days in the bone marrow and only 1 day in the periphery before maturing into an adult RBC.
  - The average RBC lives about 120 days (4 months) in the peripheral blood.
  - The average number of RBCs is 5 million/μL of blood; at 1%, the average number of reticulocytes is 50,000 cells/μL.
  - The reticulocyte count is often reflected as a percentage of RBCs; the reticulocyte index (RI) helps to determine whether the response is adequate for the degree of anemia. An RI of less than 2% is an inadequate response.

$$RI = \frac{\text{reticulocyte count} \times (\text{patient's Hct/normal Hct})}{\text{maturation factor}}$$

The maturation factor is based on the Hct:

45% = 1.0
35% = 1.5
25% = 2.0
20% = 2.5

- Under the influence of erythropoietin, the bone marrow can increase its production of reticulocytes by about 500%.

■ Classification

Various algorithms may be used to help us identify the cause of a patient's anemia. You should choose the one that works best for you in terms of enabling you to generate a logical differential diagnosis and then to narrow that diagnosis by asking the appropriate history questions, looking for the appropriate physical examination findings, and ultimately to appropriately treat a given patient's anemia.

1. The **morphologic approach** involves using the MCV to separate the anemia into one of three categories. It is the system used in this book, with a chapter devoted to each of the categories.
   - Microcytic anemias: MCV of less than 80 fL
   - Normocytic anemia: MCV of 80 to 100 fL
   - Macrocytic anemia: MCV of more than 100 fL
2. The **kinetic approach** divides the anemias based on the mechanism of reduction. In this book, the kinetic approach is used to further subdivide the normocytic anemias.
   - Decreased RBC production (hypoproliferative anemia): In this group are anemias with a low reticulocyte count, or one that is inadequate for the degree of anemia.
   - Increased RBC destruction (hyperproliferative anemias): These anemias result from destruction in the peripheral blood or from blood loss. The bone marrow responds by increasing its production of RBCs, reflected in an elevated reticulocyte count.

■ Approach to the Anemic Patient

The most important first step is to determine the severity of the anemia and the need for urgent intervention.

1. Vital signs: Look for tachycardia, orthostatic hypotension, or gross hypotension, all of which suggest a more urgent need for intervention.
2. History: Look for trauma, recent medical interventions (lines, surgeries, etc.), evidence of internal bleeding (melena, abdominal pain, hematemesis, etc.), and symptoms of anemia.

- Symptoms such as chest pain, shortness of breath, and dizziness or syncope necessitate more urgent intervention.
- Other symptoms can guide the differential diagnosis but do not require urgent intervention (pica, epigastric pain, etc.).
- A lack of symptoms suggests that the patient has had time to compensate physiologically for the anemia, which points to a more chronic course.

3. Physical examination: Look for pallor, tachycardia, tachypnea, and altered mental status, all of which suggest urgency.
   - An organ-based approach can suggest the source of anemia; of particular importance is a search for cirrhosis, spleno-megaly, jaundice, malignancy, and chronic inflammatory diseases.

4. Intervention: It is essential to thoroughly consider the pros and cons of a blood transfusion before administration; not all anemic patients should be transfused!
   - In general, patients with a history of coronary artery disease or evidence of coronary compromise (chest pain, electro-cardiographic changes) should be transfused to achieve a goal Hb level of more than 10 g/dL.
   - Patients who are asymptomatic do not require transfusion.
   - Patients with a history of sickle cell anemia should be trans-fused only when absolutely necessary; their goal Hb is their baseline Hb, which is not usually in the normal range.
   - In a nonemergent setting, it is advisable to obtain a periph-eral smear before the transfusion to better evaluate the anemia.
   - Erythropoietin has been approved for use in patients with chronic anemia resulting from chronic renal failure, human immunodeficiency virus/acquired immunodeficiency syn-drome, and certain malignancies, as well as in preoperative patients.
   - Nutrient supplementation should follow a thorough workup (see specific chapters) to identify and correct the etiology of the nutrient deficiency.

5

Microcytic Anemia

■ **BOX 5-1 Microcytic Anemias**

The microcytic anemias are straightforward and can be remembered using the mnemonic **TAILS**:

Thalassemia trait
Anemia of chronic disease
Iron-deficiency anemia
Lead poisoning
Sideroblastic anemia

Thalassemias

Adult hemoglobin is called **hemoglobin A** (Hb A) and consists of two α- and two β-globin subunits. The thalassemias are a group of disorders characterized by defective synthesis of either the α-globin or the β-globin chain. Anemia results from two mechanisms. First, there is decreased oxygen-carrying capacity because of less Hb in each red cell, which results in hypochromia and microcytosis. The second and more significant mechanism is related to clumping of the unmatched globin chains within the red cells, causing instability and membrane damage. These cells either die in the bone marrow or get trapped and destroyed in the spleen. This is known as **hemolysis,** to which the bone marrow responds by producing more red cells in the form of the larger more immature **reticulocytes.** These two mechanisms of anemia explain why thalassemia can result in either a microcytic or a macrocytic anemia.

■ β-Thalassemias

β-Thalassemias result from the defective synthesis of all or some β-globin chains resulting in a β/α ratio of less than 1. Unpaired α-chains are more toxic to the red cells than unpaired non–α-globins. These disorders are most common in the Mediterranean, Africa, and Southeast Asia.

Thalassemia Major

Homozygous for B^0 (no β-globin at all) or B^+ (few β-globin chains present), patients with thalassemia major have severe anemia first detectable at 6 to 9 months of age when fetal Hb disappears. They require regular blood transfusions, and if they survive, they have growth retardation, bony abnormalities (from massive erythropoiesis), hepatosplenomegaly (from extramedullary erythropoiesis), and hemosiderosis (from excessive absorption of iron and multiple blood transfusions). Bone marrow transplant from a human leukocyte antigen (HLA)–matched sibling is the only hope for cure.

Thalassemia Intermedia

Thalassemia intermedia includes "double heterozygotes" (B^0/B^+) and variants of the heterozygous state (B/B^0 and B/B^+) that cause more β-globin deficiency than seen in B-thalassemia minor. These patients have severe anemia but do not require regular transfusions to sustain life. Attempts to increase fetal Hb (e.g., hydroxyurea) are variably effective.

Thalassemia Minor

Patients with minor are heterozygous with one normal β-globin gene and either a B^0 or a B^+. The B/B^0 state is referred to as **B-thal trait** and is thought to confer some protection against falciparum malaria. Patients with B/B^+ are referred to as **silent carriers.** In either case, these patients are asymptomatic and do not require treatment. Microcytosis, hypochromia, and even mild anemia may be present. Consider genetic counseling for these individuals and their partners if they are planning to conceive.

■ α-Thalassemias

α-Thalassemias are the defective synthesis of all or some α-globin chains; note that four genes code for the α-globin chains, so the degree of severity depends on the number of genes affected.

Hydrops Fetalis

Hydrops fetalis is caused by the deletion of all four α-globin genes, leaving fetal red blood cells (RBCs) with aggregates of γ-globins, which form tetramers (**Hb Barts**). The high oxygen affinity of these tetramers results in tissue anoxia and intrauterine fetal death.

Hemoglobin H Disease

In Hb H disease, three of four α-globin genes are deleted, resulting in aggregates of β-globins known as **Hb H.** The disease occurs mainly in Asians and the symptoms of anemia may appear out of proportion to the measured hemoglobin because the Hb H has a high oxygen affinity (thus, it delivers less oxygen to the tissues).

α-Thalassemia Trait

The α-thalassemia trait is caused by the deletion of two α-globin genes, which results in an asymptomatic state, with minimal to no anemia.

Silent Carrier State

The silent carrier state is when the deletion of one α-globin gene results in an unappreciable reduction in α-globins; thus, these patients are neither symptomatic nor anemic.

Anemia of Chronic Disease

Anemia of chronic disease (ACD) is a type of anemia that may be microcytic or normocytic and is thought to result from impaired mobilization of iron from iron stores in the production of RBCs. There is also inadequate erythropoietin production (via cytokine interleukin-1 [IL-1]) and insensitivity of the red cell precursors to erythropoietin (via cytokines interferon-γ [IFN-γ] and tumor necrosis factor [TNF]). ACD is related to chronic inflammatory diseases that fall into the following three categories:

1. Chronic infections: osteomyelitis, endocarditis, tuberculosis
2. Chronic autoimmune disorders: lupus, rheumatoid arthritis
3. Malignancy: lymphomas, some carcinomas

This anemia is characterized by a normal to elevated ferritin level, low total iron binding capacity (TIBC), normal iron saturation, and low to normal serum iron concentration. The reticulocyte count is inadequate for the degree of anemia.

Iron-Deficiency Anemia

Anemia resulting from iron deficiency does not appear until there is significant depletion of iron stores (Box 5-2). Inadequate Hb synthesis results in microcytosis. Clinical signs and symptoms specific to iron deficiency include koilonychia (spoon nails), atrophic glossitis, alopecia, esophageal web (Plummer-Vinson syndrome), and pica (a craving for nonfood items such as chalk, clay, or ice). This anemia is characterized by low ferritin level, low serum iron concentration, elevated TIBC, low iron saturation (<15%), and low reticulocyte count. In mixed disorders (e.g., renal failure plus upper gastrointestinal [GI] tract bleed), a low iron saturation is helpful in establishing the presence of iron-deficiency anemia.

The most common causes of iron deficiency differ depending on age, sex, and geographic region and are discussed in more detail in the following sections.

■ BOX 5-2 All about Iron

- Men need a daily intake of 5–10 mg of iron; women need 7–20 mg daily.
- 80% of the body's iron is found in hemoglobin (3 g).
- 20% is in storage (800 mg) in the form of ferritin or hemosiderin.
- Transferrin, synthesized in the liver, is the iron transporter and is usually 33% saturated (i.e., total iron binding capacity of iron is three times that of transferrin).
- Dietary iron must be released from apoproteins by gastric acid to be absorbed.
- 25% of heme-bound iron (from meat) is absorbed, whereas only 1% to 2% of inorganic iron is absorbed.
- Ascorbic acid (vitamin C) enhances the absorption of inorganic iron.

Thus, after a 5-g loss of hemoglobin, the body needs about 1 g of iron; 325 mg of $FeSO_4$ three times a day will result in absorption of 1% or 3 mg three times a day (i.e., 9 mg daily). With a fixed daily loss of 1 mg of iron, it will take about 125 days of therapy to replace the lost iron.

■ Chronic Gastrointestinal Blood Loss

Chronic GI tract blood loss is the most important cause among postmenopausal women and adult men in developed countries. Black tarry stools (melena) and symptoms of postprandial epigastric pain suggest upper GI tract blood loss, whereas bright red blood in the stool points toward lower GI tract bleeds. Hookworm and pinworm infestations of the GI tract commonly cause iron-deficiency anemia in developing countries.

■ Other Chronic Blood Loss

The most common cause of iron deficiency in menstruating women is gynecologic blood loss. In adults, also consider the urinary tract.

■ Increased Requirements

Growing infants, children, and menstruating adolescents have greater iron requirements than the average adult. Pregnant women are at risk because they tend to start pregnancy with depleted iron stores as a result of past menses.

■ Dietary Insufficiency

Dietary insufficiency is rare in developed countries except among the poor, the elderly (poor diet), and vegetarians (inorganic iron is less absorbable than that found in meat).

■ Impaired Absorption

Chronic diarrhea and steatorrhea increase transit time through the small bowel. Gastrectomy results in decreased stomach acid, which is required for iron absorption.

- **Celiac sprue** is the most common inherited form of iron deficiency and should be considered in patients who do not respond to iron replacement. Patients can present at any time from childhood to adolescence and may have an intermittent course with exacerbations characterized by diarrhea, weight loss, and nutrient deficiencies. Antiendomysial antibodies are sensitive and specific for this disease, but small bowel biopsy (revealing flattened duodenal/jejunal villi) is required to establish the diagnosis. Dietary restriction of gluten (found in wheat, barley, rice, and oats) is an important part of therapy.
- Excess phosphates, tannates (sodas, teas), carbonates, and oxalates may inhibit iron absorption.

Lead Poisoning

Lead is found in paints, batteries, plumbing fixtures, and improperly glazed ceramics. It inhibits ferrochelatase and aminolevulinic acid (ALA) dehydratase, which are necessary in the production of Hb. In addition to anemia, signs and symptoms of lead exposure include irritability, neurocognitive decline, abdominal pain, renal impairment, peripheral neuropathy, and lead lines (dark lines at the gingival-tooth border). Serum and urine ALA levels are elevated, as is erythrocyte protoporphyrin, in the setting of lead intoxication. Treatment with chelation (CaEDTA) is recommended for adults with serum lead levels of more than 80 μg/dL or more than 60 μg/dL with signs and/or symptoms. However, because lead is stored in bone, conditions of bone resorption (e.g., hyperthyroidism, osteoporosis, and pregnancy) may release lead absorbed years earlier, a scenario whose clinical significance is unclear.

The peripheral smear may show basophilic stippling of RBCs (dark blue dots).

Sideroblastic Anemia

Sideroblastic anemia results from an impaired incorporation of intracellular iron into the heme molecule. RBC precursors with excess iron are called **sideroblasts.** Basophilic stippling may be seen on the peripheral smear. Sideroblastic anemia may be seen in the myelodysplastic syndromes, which affect older adults and are generally preneoplastic.

Serum iron may be derated, or all indices may be generally within the normal reference range in sideroblastic anemia.

Normocytic Anemia

For anemias with a normal **mean corpuscular volume** (MCV), we can use the reticulocyte count to determine whether the disorder results from decreased production by the bone marrow, increased destruction in the peripheral blood system, or acute blood loss (not sufficient to cause iron deficiency) (Figure 6-1).

HYPOPROLIFERATIVE ANEMIAS

Hypoproliferative anemias result in anemia without an effective bone marrow response. If two or more cell lines are affected (i.e., anemia with low platelet and/or low leukocyte counts), a bone marrow biopsy must be pursued to rule out an infiltrative/infectious process in the marrow.

Pure Red Cell Aplasia

Among adults, pure red cell aplasia (PRCA) is an acquired disorder and can be treatable.

- **Acute Parvovirus B19** infection can cause PRCA in the setting of underlying hemolytic anemias (e.g., sickle cell) and usually resolves once the infection clears.
- **Chronic Parvovirus B19** infection, usually seen in immunodeficient patients, responds to intravenous immunoglobulin (IVIg); look for giant pronormoblasts in the bone marrow biopsy specimen.
- The congenital form of PRCA, **Diamond-Blackfan syndrome,** responds to glucocorticoid therapy. One third of these children will have a congenital anomaly (e.g., absent thumb, small stature, cleft palate, and heart disease).
- Transient erythroblastopenia of childhood is a rare disorder of unknown etiology affecting children at around age 2 years (later than Diamond-Blackfan syndrome) and resolving spontaneously usually after a few months.

Aplastic Anemia

- A rare disorder with an incidence of only two per million in the west and six per million in Southeast Asia.

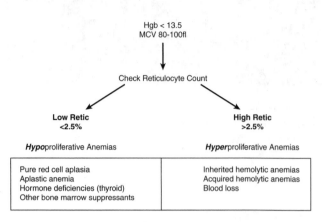

Figure 6-1 • Hypoproliferative anemias vs. hyperproliferative anemias

- There is a bimodal age distribution (young adulthood and elderly).
- Most cases of acquired aplastic anemia are caused by T-cell–mediated destruction of hematopoietic cells in the bone marrow; specifically, interferon-γ (IFN-g) is thought to be responsible for the apoptosis of CD34+ cells (stem cells).
- The peripheral smear typically shows reduction in all three cell lines with a normal to elevated MCV.
- Grossly, the cellular component of bone marrow is replaced by fat.
- It is thought that an inciting event initiates the process, such as viral illnesses (hepatitis, mononucleosis) or chemical exposure (benzene, chloramphenicol, indomethacin).
- The need for treatment is based on severity of cytopenia; long-term immunosuppression with antithymocyte globulin (ATG) plus cyclosporine or high-dose cyclophosphamide is effective in more than 75% of patients.
- Bone marrow transplantation is still considered optimal therapy, provided that a human leukocyte antigen (HLA)–matched sibling donor can be identified.
- About 25% of these patients have the **paroxysmal nocturnal hemoglobinuria** (PNH) mutation (deficient CD55 or CD59); the significance of the "overlapping" of these two syndromes is unclear.

Hormonal Influences

■ Erythropoietin

Anemia in patients with chronic renal insufficiency is due to inadequate production of erythropoietin by the failing kidneys, usually once the glomerular filtration rate (GFR) falls below 30 mL/min. Recombinant human erythropoietin has improved the treatment of this anemia. These patients must have adequate iron, folate, and vitamin B_{12} for the bone marrow to respond to the exogenous stimulus. Also, beware that blood loss in combination with chronic disease may yield a falsely elevated ferritin level and iron saturation (consider working up iron-deficiency anemia in patients with renal failure with a ferritin level of less than 100 and saturation of less than 20%).

■ Androgens

One of the reasons that the normal range of hemoglobin (Hb) is higher in men than in women is that testosterone promotes erythropoiesis in the bone marrow.

■ Thyroid Hormone

Various comorbid conditions can contribute to anemia in patients with hypothyroidism. Menorrhagia, for example, is more common in these patients. In addition, 10% of patients with hypothyroidism also have pernicious anemia. However, hypothyroidism by itself seems to cause a mild normocytic or macrocytic anemia that improves once the deficiency is treated.

■ Parathyroid Hormone

In hyperparathyroidism, renal erythropoietin may be inhibited because of the toxic effects of hypercalcemia on the kidneys.

■ Addison Disease

Patients with Addison disease, once rehydrated, are often anemic with inadequate bone marrow stimulation resulting from reduced androgen and steroid synthesis.

Marrow Infiltration/Fibrosis

The bone marrow may fail to increase production of blood cells as a result of infectious, infiltrative, or fibrotic processes such as tuberculosis, sarcoidosis, lymphomas, metastatic neoplasms, or idiopathic myelofibrosis.

HYPERPROLIFERATIVE ANEMIAS

Hyperproliferative anemias occur because of processes in the periphery—loss of red cells through bleeding or destruction in the intravascular or extravascular compartments. We can also say that in these anemias, the lifetime of all or some of the red cells is reduced. The healthy bone marrow attempts to replace the red cells by increasing production, which is manifested by an increased reticulocyte count. In the case of hemolysis, or peripheral destruction of red cells, other laboratory findings include an elevated indirect bilirubin and lactate dehydrogenase (LDH), which are due to heme breakdown and red cell lysis, respectively. Free heme becomes bound by circulating haptoglobin, reducing its serum level. Beware: These laboratory findings can also indicate internal bleeding, so be sure to check stool, urine, and possible iatrogenic causes! Also note that with brisk reticulocytosis, the MCV may be elevated in any of the hemolytic disorders.

Inherited Hemolytic Anemias

The inherited hemolytic anemias include disorders of defective Hb synthesis, red cell membrane defects, and red cell enzyme deficiencies. A mnemonic for the inherited hemolytic anemias follows in Box 6-1. For a thorough discussion of the thalassemias, please refer to the section Microcytic Anemia.

■ Red Cell Enzyme Deficiencies

Glucose-6-Phosphate Dehydrogenase Deficiency

Glucose-6-phosphate dehydrogenase (G6PD) deficiency is a disorder that affects about 400 million people, especially in tropical Africa, the Middle East, subtropical Asia, and the Mediterranean. It is believed to protect against malaria by promoting red blood cell (RBC) destruction in the setting of oxidative stressors (such as infection). There is considerable variability in the specific genetic defect, but the enzyme is located on the X chromosome, so the disorder predominantly affects men. Precipitants of oxidized Hb in RBCs may be visible on the peripheral blood smear; these are known as **Heinz bodies.**

■ BOX 6-1 Inherited Hemolytic Anemias

The inherited hemolytic anemias can **BE PASS**ed on in families:
  β-thalassemia
  Enzyme deficiencies (glucose-6-phosphate dehydrogenase, pyruvate kinase)
  Porphyria
  α-thalassemia
  Sickle cell anemia
  Spherocytosis (membrane defects)

■ BOX 6-2 Agents/Conditions Known to Promote Hemolytic Episodes in G6PD-Deficient Patients

<u>D</u>oxorubicin	<u>M</u>oth balls
<u>I</u>nfections	<u>A</u>cidosis
<u>V</u>itamin K	<u>N</u>itrofurantoin
<u>A</u>ntimalarials: primaquines, dapsone	
<u>S</u>ulfonamides: sulfamethoxazole (Bactrim)	
Fava beans	

Triggers of hemolysis in G6PD deficiency are listed in Box 6.2. Think of "Mediterranean **DIVA MAN,** Saul, turning yellow eating fava beans."

Pyruvate Kinase Deficiency

Pyruvate kinase (PK) deficiency is an autosomal recessive disorder that affects the glycolytic pathway in the RBC and can cause a moderate to severe hemolytic anemia. There may be partial resolution with splenectomy.

Triosephosphate Isomerase Deficiency

Much less common than PK deficiency, triosephosphate isomerase deficiency also affects the glycolytic pathway. In addition to hemolytic anemia, patients can present with recurrent infections (because the enzyme is also lacking in leukocytes) and progressive neurologic dysfunction, usually in childhood.

■ Porphyrias

- **Congenital erythropoietic porphyria** (CEP): This autosomal recessive form of porphyria results in reduced levels of urosynthase, an enzyme involved in the synthesis of heme. Unmetabolized porphyrins build up in bone, red cells, urine, and feces. Patients usually have a chronic hemolytic anemia with splenomegaly. Severe photosensitivity is characteristic, with disfiguring bullae and vesicles on sun-exposed skin.
- Hemolytic anemia is not a characteristic finding in the other types of porphyria.

■ Sickle Cell Anemia

- Sickle cell anemia results from an autosomal recessive disorder, the gene for which is carried in approximately 8% of African Americans and in about 2% of persons of Mediterranean descent.
- The mutation involves the substitution of valine for glutamic acid at position 6 in the β-globin chain.

- This results in Hb S, which when deoxygenated, polymerizes (Hb Ss aggregate with each other, but less so with other types of β-globins) and deforms the RBC.
- The degree of anemia and response to hypoxia depends on whether the patient inherits a mutant globin gene from the other parent as well.
- The definitive diagnosis is made by Hb electrophoresis, although the presence of irreversibly sickled cells with anemia (hematocrit [Hct] usually 20% to 25%) and hemolysis (reticulocyte count 15% to 20%) strongly suggests the diagnosis.

Homozygous (SS)

Patients who are homozygous inherit the defective gene for the valine substitution on the β-globin from both parents. Nearly all of the Hb in their RBCs is Hb S, with variable amounts of persistent Hb F. Conditions that increase the interaction between intracellular Hb S increase the tendency to sickle; for example, dehydration shrinks cells, allowing Hb S chains to get closer to each other. Interestingly, patients with coexisting α-thalassemia have less severe disease because of decreased overall production of Hb.

- Pain crises (a.k.a., vaso-occlusive crises) are the hallmark of the disease and may affect bone, lung, liver, brain, spleen, and the penis. Treatment involves hydration, analgesia, and ruling out other etiologies (infection, aseptic necrosis). Hydroxyurea has been shown to decrease the number of pain crises.
- Children may present with **dactylitis,** a painful swelling of the hands and feet.
- **Splenic sequestration crises,** most common in infancy, involve massive RBC sequestration by an enlarging spleen, which may lead to hypovolemia and shock (consider transfusion followed by splenectomy).
- **Acute chest syndrome** is suggested by dyspnea with lung infiltrates that are due to sequestration of red cells in the pulmonary circulation (treat as soon as possible with exchange transfusion).
- **Infection** with encapsulated organisms, likely due to splenic dysfunction (patients usually autoinfarct the spleen during childhood), is common. Patients should be offered immunizations against *Streptococcus pneumoniae, Haemophilus influenzae,* and *Neisseria meningitidis.*
- Chronic hemolysis predisposes to gallstones and renal failure.
- Acute/chronic **osteomyelitis** should always be considered in patients with bony complaints; *Staphylococcus aureus* is the most common etiology, but these patients are at increased risk of *Salmonella typhi.*

- There is also increased risk of aplastic anemia due to infection with Parvovirus B19; look for anemia with a very low reticulocyte count.

Heterozygous (AS)

Patients who are heterozygous produce about 40% Hb S and 60% Hb A. Hb A is much less likely to aggregate with Hb S, so these patients do not sickle (unless they are exposed to severe hypoxia), and they have neither anemia nor hemolysis. This state is also referred to as **sickle cell trait.**

Hemoglobin SC (Compound Heterozygotes)

Patients who are considered compound heterozygotes inherit the Hb S gene and another mutant β-globin known as Hb C. They have approximately equal amounts of each type of Hb in their RBCs. Hb C does polymerize with Hb S, though to a lesser extent than Hb S to itself, so these patients suffer anemia and hemolysis to a lesser degree than homozygotes for Hb S.

These patients suffer fewer pain crises but can have severe complications including retinal damage and blindness, aseptic necrosis of the femoral heads, and pulmonary syndromes.

Sickle Cell Thalassemia (Compound Heterozygotes)

Patients with sickle cell thalassemia inherit the sickle cell gene from one parent and the β-thalassemia from the other. They produce predominantly Hb S and thus are clinically indistinguishable from homozygotes.

■ Red Cell Membrane Disorders

In red cell membrane disorders, defects in the red cell membrane allow early death in the peripheral blood.

Congenital Spherocytosis

Congenital spherocytosis occurs in about 1 in 1000 to 4500 births and involves defects in the membrane anchoring proteins spectrin and ankyrin.

- The defects are usually inherited in an autosomal dominant pattern.
- On the peripheral smear, these cells lack central pallor.
- Because of their decreased surface area, they are unable to take in free water and lyse more readily in hypoosmolar sodium chloride (osmotic fragility test).
- Patients may exhibit jaundice and anemia, especially during episodes of trauma, infection, or other stressors, but generally, the bone marrow can maintain a normal Hb.
- Like all patients with chronic hemolysis, these patients are at increased risk of pigmented gallstones. Patients with gallstones

should have the gallbladder and spleen removed simultaneously, because leaving the spleen behind allows continued hemolysis, thereby increasing the risk of intrahepatic cholelithiasis.

- **Splenomegaly** is usually present as the rigid spherocytes become trapped on their way through the sinusoids.
- **Splenectomy** corrects the anemia; beware of accessory spleens if anemia recurs postoperatively.

Hereditary Elliptocytosis

With a similar incidence to congenital spherocytosis (about 1 in 4000), hereditary elliptocytosis is also an autosomal dominant disorder involving deficient spectrin. These cells deform during passage through the spleen and microcirculation but are unable to revert to their normal shape. Hemolysis is usually only mild; splenectomy is effective in cases of severe anemia.

Hereditary Stomacytosis

Hereditary stomacytosis is an autosomal dominant disorder that is more rare, with cup-shaped RBCs that usually manifest slits of central pallor on peripheral smear.

Acquired Hemolytic Anemias

- Thinking of red cells getting **SPLIT** is a helpful mnemonic (Box 6-3)

■ Splenic Sequestration

- An enlarged spleen can entrap RBCs and reticulocytes, resulting in shortened red cell survival.
- Look for an elevated reticulocyte count, normal to mildly elevated bilirubin concentration, and underlying causes of splenomegaly (e.g., evidence of cirrhosis).

■ BOX 6-3 Acquired Hemolytic Anemias—*SPLIT*

Splenic sequestration
Paroxysmal nocturnal hemoglobinuria
Lysis by toxins/infections
 • Metals, bites, malaria
Immune mediated
 • Warm/cold autoimmune
 • Isoimmune
Trauma
 • Macrovascular (valves)
 • Microvascular (disseminated intravascular coagulation, thrombotic thrombocytopenic purpura)

■ Paroxysmal Nocturnal Hemoglobinuria

- Paroxysmal nocturnal hemoglobinuria is an acquired mutation in the X-linked pigA gene, resulting in deficient membrane proteins **CD55** and **CD59.** This deficiency renders RBCs more susceptible to lysis by complement, especially at lower blood pH levels (as occurs at night—hence, the nighttime hemoglobinuria—although this finding is not consistent).
- Patients have varying degrees of anemia and hemolysis; leukopenia and thrombocytopenia are common and are thought to result from defective hematopoiesis (rather than peripheral destruction, although these cells are also deficient in CD55 and CD59).
- The diagnosis is made by flow cytometry for the presence of CD55/59; the Ham test for acid-induced hemolysis is no longer standard.
- 40% of patients with PNH will have venous thrombosis, often in the intra-abdominal veins; they may also have symptomatic anemia, pancytopenia, or jaundice from hemolysis.

■ Lysis by Toxins/Infections

Various environmental exposures can directly lyse RBCs:
- Metals (e.g., copper salts)
- Snake bites, spider bites (brown recluse)
- Heat (e.g., severe burns)
- Infections (e.g., malaria, babesiosis, *Bartonella*, and bacteremia with *Staphylococcus*, *S. pneumoniae*, and *Escherichia coli*)

■ Immune Mediated

The autoimmune hemolytic anemias (warm and cold) are rare disorders, affecting approximately 1 to 3 persons per 100,000 per year. They involve immunoglobulin G (IgG) or immunoglobulin M (IgM) antibodies directed against antigens on the patient's own RBCs. *Alloimmunity* refers to antibodies directed against foreign antigens on transfused or newborn RBCs.

Warm Autoimmune Hemolytic Anemia

Warm autoimmune hemolytic anemia is the more common form of autoimmune hemolysis and involves IgG antibodies, with or without complement (C3), which have their optimal affinity for RBCs at 37°C. Usually, Fc receptors on splenic macrophages bind the IgG-covered RBCs and destroy them, a process termed extravascular hemolysis. The etiology is usually related to an underlying disorder (see later discussion) but may be idiopathic. The incidence increases after age 40 years and women are affected twice as frequently as men.

- Look for signs of hemolysis with elevated indirect bilirubin level, elevated reticulocyte count, low haptoglobin, hemoglobinuria, and a positive direct Coombs test result (in >95% of cases). The peripheral smear will show spherocytes (as opposed to the schistocytes seen in traumatic hemolysis), resulting from partial destruction of RBCs in the spleen.
- Patients typically have an indolent course, with nonspecific symptoms related to anemia, as well as jaundice and splenomegaly.
- Conditions conferring increased risk include autoimmune diseases like lupus and rheumatoid arthritis, lymphoproliferative disorders such as lymphoma, Hodgkin disease, and Waldenström macroglobinemia, and viral illnesses such as human immunodeficiency virus, and Epstein-Barr virus.
- Prednisone (1–2 mg/kg/day) is the mainstay of therapy, with splenectomy reserved for steroid-refractory patients. In some patients, symptoms still recur and require long-term steroids or other immunosuppressive agents (e.g., cyclophosphamide).

Cold Autoimmune Hemolytic Anemia

Cold autoimmune hemolytic anemia is a type of hemolysis that is mediated by IgM antibodies, which have their optimal affinity for RBCs at less than normal body temperature. Splenic macrophages do not have Fc receptors for IgM, so hemolysis is usually mediated by complement and occurs within the vasculature.

- Look for a mild anemia with mild reticulocytosis and clumping of RBCs at room temperature.
- Patients may complain of acrocyanosis in the distal extremities in cold temperatures.
- Secondary causes include infection with *Mycoplasma pneumoniae* and mononucleosis (transient cold agglutinins), as well as underlying lymphoproliferative disorders such as lymphoma and benign monoclonal gammopathy.
- Steroids and splenectomy are usually ineffective; generally, the problem resolves with treatment of the underlying disorder.

Drug-Induced Hemolytic Anemia

Drug-induced hemolytic anemia can result from a process identical to warm autoimmune hemolytic anemia or from binding of the drug or its metabolites to the RBC, forming a complex (haptene) to which the body develops antibodies.

- α-Methyldopa induces an IgG antibody to Rh antigens on self-RBCs. The Coombs test result is positive and may remain positive even long after the drug is withdrawn; spherocytes are visible on the blood smear.

- Penicillin binds to RBCs, inducing an IgG antibody to the haptene—hence, resulting in a positive direct Coombs test result; the peripheral smear reveals spherocytes and there is usually a mild hemolysis, which resolves on removal of the drug.
- Quinidine and sulfa drugs bind less tightly to RBCs and usually induce IgM antibodies, which fix complement, causing a positive direct Coombs test result with C3 only. The indirect Coombs test result is positive only if the drug is added to the reaction. Hemolysis resolves upon removal of the drug.

Alloimmune Hemolytic Anemia

Alloimmune hemolytic anemia results from antibodies against foreign antigens on transfused RBCs or in newborns in whom maternal antibodies react against fetal Rh (erythroblastosis fetalis).

■ Traumatic Hemolysis

In traumatic hemolysis, RBCs can be damaged as they pass through the macrovasculature and microvasculature.

- Macrovascular trauma: About 10% of patients with cardiac valves have evidence of RBC damage with fragmented RBCs (schistocytes) on the peripheral smear.
- Microvascular trauma: Fibrin deposition from intravascular coagulation can cause sheer stress, resulting in schistocytes on the peripheral smear. This process is known as **microangiopathic hemolytic anemia** and occurs in disseminated intravascular coagulation, thrombotic thrombocytopenic purpura, hemolytic uremic syndrome, and HELLP (hemolysis, elevated liver enzymes, low platelets) syndrome. For a thorough review of the microangiopathic hemolytic anemias, please see the section on thrombocytopenia.

Acute Blood Loss

The renal response to hypoxia is to increase secretion of erythropoietin. In normal bone marrow with adequate iron stores, reticulocytosis will become evident in the first 48 hours but will not be maximal until 7 to 10 days after significant loss of blood.

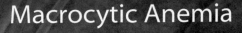

Macrocytic Anemia

The macrocytic anemias can be divided into the megaloblastic and nonmegaloblastic subtypes. In the megaloblastic anemias, nutritional deficits hinder DNA synthesis while the cells' cytoplasmic proteins continue to mature, resulting in asynchronous hematopoiesis. The bone marrow becomes hypercellular in response to the peripheral anemia. The bone marrow is not hypercellular in nonmegaloblastic anemias.

Megaloblastic Anemias

■ Vitamin B_{12} Deficiency

- Without vitamin B_{12}, nuclear mitosis in the developing cells of the bone marrow is inhibited, resulting in large red blood cells (RBCs) with mature cytoplasmic proteins but with immature nuclei.
  - These cells often die in the bone marrow, releasing intracellular lactate dehydrogenase (LDH), which leaks into the bloodstream.
  - The cells that do emerge from the bone marrow appear on the peripheral smear as large RBCs with occasional nucleated RBCs.
  - Because B_{12} is necessary for DNA synthesis in all cells, thrombocytopenia and leukopenia may also be present.
  - Classically, the smear also reveals hypersegmented neutrophils (granulocytes with more than five to six nuclei).
- B_{12} is also involved in the production of succinyl coenzyme A (Krebs cycle), so its deficiency leads to elevated levels of methylmalonic acid (MMA), a precursor in that reaction.
  - The elevated MMA may be responsible for abnormal neuronal lipid production and the neurologic deficits attributable to B_{12} deficiency. Neurologic complaints can range from dorsal column symptoms to neurocognitive decline.
  - The serum MMA can be helpful in distinguishing B_{12} from folate deficiency and in diagnosing early B_{12} deficiency in patients with borderline macrocytosis or neurologic deficits without anemia.

- The most common cause of B_{12} deficiency is **pernicious anemia** (PA), an autoimmune condition in which antiparietal cell or anti-intrinsic factor antibodies prevent absorption of B_{12} from the gastrointestinal (GI) tract.
  - The antibodies can be detected in about three fourths of patients with PA. The destruction of parietal cells is thought to results in the failure to secrete intrinsic factor and the autoantibodies are simply markers of parietal cell destruction, rather than its cause.
  - Endoscopy may reveal chronic atrophic gastritis with a higher than normal pH level.
  - These patients are at increased risk of gastric cancer and are more likely to suffer from other autoimmune disorders, such as thyroiditis.
- Other causes of B_{12} deficiency include decreased dietary intake, decreased ileal absorption of B_{12}, parasitic infection, and other GI disorders.
  - Generally, only strict vegans are at risk of inadequate intake.
  - Even patients who stop consuming animal products will have adequate B_{12} stores for up to 5 years.
  - Patients with diseases of ileum, such as Crohn disease, or who have had ileal resections are at risk of developing the deficiency.
  - GI tract infection with the fish tapeworm *Diphyllobothrium latum* has also been implicated in preventing B_{12} absorption.

■ Folic Acid Deficiency

- Since the 1998 the United States has mandated the fortification of staple foods like bread and cereal with folate, thus reducing the incidence of folate deficiency and associated congenital neural tube defects.
- Folate deficiency causes the same spectrum of laboratory and blood smear findings as B_{12} deficiency but does not increase the serum MMA level.
- Both vitamins are part of the DNA synthesis pathway, and a deficiency of either will result in elevated homocysteine levels, a precursor in that enzyme cascade.
- Physicians should beware of masking B_{12} deficiency by treating a macrocytic anemia with folate alone, because the neurologic deficits related to the insufficient B_{12} can progress in spite of the normalized mean corpuscular volume (MCV).

Nonmegaloblastic Anemia

■ Drugs/Toxins

- It is essential to rule out iatrogenic causes of macrocytosis before pursuing an extensive workup of organic causes. The agents that cause macrocytosis usually impair DNA metabolism. Here are the more common examples:
  - AZT (you can confirm compliance with human immunodeficiency virus [HIV] meds by checking the MCV!)
  - Methotrexate
  - Azathioprine
  - Thalidomide
  - Dilantin
  - Alcohol

■ Liver Disease

- Patients with liver disease are susceptible to anemia from blood loss, splenomegaly, and nutritional deficiencies.
- However, cirrhotic patients can also exhibit a macrocytic anemia that is thought to be related to abnormal lipid deposition in the RBC membrane.
  - These cells may be visible on the peripheral blood smear as burr cells, and their early death in the spleen resembles a mild hemolytic anemia.

■ Reticulocytosis

- Reticulocytes are RBC precursors that usually live 1 to 2 days in the peripheral blood before becoming mature RBCs.
- They are slightly larger and bluer (more basophilic) than mature RBCs, and they lack central pallor.
- In conditions such as hemolysis, an elevated MCV may represent the larger number and longer survival of reticulocytes in the peripheral blood.

■ Myelodysplastic Syndrome

- Myelodysplastic syndrome (MDS) is an interesting family of bone marrow disorders that results almost uniformly in large RBCs.
- Patients are often elderly and, in addition to anemia, usually exhibit decreased bone marrow production of neutrophils and/or platelets.
- Older patients with macrocytosis in whom B_{12} and folate deficiencies have been ruled out should be evaluated for MDS with a bone marrow biopsy.

8 Thrombocytopenia

■ Etiology

- Three major categories are as follows:
  - Destruction
  - Bone marrow failure
  - Sequestration
- Three minor categories are as follows:
  - Dilutional
  - Pregnancy
  - Inherited
- EDTA clumping: pseudothrombocytopenia

Destruction

- Thrombotic thrombocytopenic purpura (TTP)
- Heparin-induced thrombocytopenia (HIT)
- Idiopathic thrombocytopenia purpura (ITP)
- Drug/radiation induced
- Post-transfusion purpura
- Autoimmune: Evans syndrome (concomitant ITP and autoimmune hemolytic anemia), thyroid (Graves disease or Hashimoto thyroiditis), lupus
- Lupus anticoagulant
- Infection: hepatitis C, human immunodeficiency virus (HIV)
- Disseminated intravascular coagulation (DIC)
- Large hemangiomas: Kasabach-Merritt syndrome
- Heart disease
- Cardiopulmonary bypass

Bone Marrow Failure

- Ethanol abuse
- Nutritional deficiencies
- Marrow failure: aplastic anemia
- Marrow infiltration: metastatic carcinoma, lymphoma, leukemia
- Drugs
- Radiation
- Inherited

Sequestration

- Hypersplenism

Dilutional
- Massive transfusion

Pregnancy
- Incidental
- ITP
- HELLP syndrome: hemolysis, elevated liver enzymes, low platelets

■ History
- Evaluate life-threatening causes first, such as TTP, HIT, or DIC.
- Consider heparin or low-molecular-weight heparin exposure.
- Compile a medication list, with emphasis on new medications.
- Consider recent transfusions.
- Inquire about recent infections.
- Evaluate for heart disease or recent cardiopulmonary bypass.
- Inquire regarding alcohol and drug exposure, specifically cocaine.
- In a woman, consider pregnancy.
- Investigate previous episodes of thrombocytopenia, including during childhood.
- Ask the patient regarding HIV and hepatitis C risk factors.
- Consider autoimmune diseases

■ Laboratory Evaluation
- First always look at peripheral smear: Evaluate for large platelets, concurrent anemia, and white blood cell differential.
- Evaluate for concurrent anemia, if microangiopathic hemolytic anemia (MAHA) on smear; seriously consider TTP.
- Test for hepatitis C and HIV, lupus anticoagulant, direct Coombs test, routine chemistry panel, DIC panel, and blood cultures if appropriate.
- Bone marrow biopsy and aspirate if bone marrow failure is highly suspected.

■ Physical Examination
- Signs of infection: fever, respiratory, urinary, or dermatologic signs
- Lymphadenopathy, hepatosplenomegaly
- Petechiae, purpura, and wet purpura (oral mucosa bleeding or eyelid petechiae)
- Thrombosis in legs and/or lungs
- Decreased oxygen saturation or respiratory alkalosis; signs of pulmonary embolism
- Painful heparin injection sites
- Heart murmurs
- Wasting, cachexia: signs of malignancy or advanced HIV

PLATELET DESTRUCTION THROMBOCYTOPENIA

- Is the most urgent consideration.
- May necessitate treatment urgently.
- Review smear in timely fashion.

Thrombotic Thrombocytopenic Purpura

- Devastating disease without prompt recognition

■ Criteria

- Only two diagnostic criteria are required for the diagnosis of TTP:
  1. Thrombocytopenia: usually very low (10,000 to 25,000 μl platelets)
  2. MAHA: visualized on peripheral blood smear; fragmented red blood cells (RBCs), helmet cells, schistocytes, and occasional nucleated RBCs.
- Previously, the diagnosis of TTP was made by a pentad of features: thrombocytopenia, MAHA, fever, renal abnormalities, and neurologic symptoms.
- However, when and if the patient has all five, he or she will be seriously ill.
- Patients need to be diagnosed before developing all five symptoms of the pentad.
- Thus, the dyad (thrombocytopenia and MAHA) is sufficient criteria for TTP (Box 8-1).

■ Clinical Manifestations

- Neurologic symptoms: headache, confusion, coma
- Renal abnormalities: proteinuria, hematuria, and renal failure more likely to be seen in hemolytic uremic syndrome
- Fever: approximately 25% of the time and nonspecific
- Abdominal pain: can be the presenting symptom of TTP
- Thrombotic and hemorrhagic complications
- Symptoms from low platelet counts are rare; usually no purpura

■ Laboratory Tests

- Very low platelet counts that drop fast.
- Platelet counts can be spuriously high because of RBC fragmentation counted by automated particle counters.

■ BOX 8-1 Thrombotic Thrombocytopenic Purpura: Dyad

Thrombocytopenia and microangiopathic hemolytic anemia are all that are needed to make the diagnosis of thrombotic thrombocytopenic purpura.

- Leukocytosis.
- Lactate dehydrogenase (LDH) is almost always elevated into the thousands range.
- Elevated bilirubin; indirect bilirubin is the predominant component indicative of hemolysis.
- Normal coagulation profile.

■ Pathophysiology

- Disorder of a deficiency of ADAMTS-13 activity, either congenital or acquired.
- ADAMTS-13 is a metalloprotease that cleaves the peptide bond of a mature von Willebrand factor (vWf).
- A deficient protease allows vWfs to become unusually large and sticky in the circulation.
- Under shear stress, the sticky factors bind platelets and form thrombi.
- RBCs are passively sheared when traversing blood vessels occluded by platelets and unusually large vWf thrombi.

■ Treatment

- Plasma exchange should be instituted immediately.
- Involves placing a large-bore vascular catheter for exchange.
- Patients should not receive platelet transfusions, unless absolutely required; platelets will add "fuel to the fire."
- Daily plasma exchange with fresh frozen plasma or cryosupernatant, not cryoprecipitate (as this contains vWfs).
- Continue until platelet counts normalize and patient improves clinically.
- LDH normalizes by process of exchange, so it is not the best test to follow.
- Function of exchange: Remove vWf multimers and platelets and replace missing proteases.
- 90% of cases resolve with appropriate treatment.

Heparin-Induced Thrombocytopenia

■ Classification

- Two types: Nonimmune and immune mediated

Nonimmune

- Heparin binds platelets, resulting in a transient, benign, self-limiting thrombocytopenia, even if continued on heparin.
- Platelet count is generally only slightly reduced.

Immune
- Generation of immunoglobulin G (IgG) antibodies to heparin and platelet factor-4 complexes, which results in platelet activation.

■ **Clinical Manifestations**
- High morbidity without prompt recognition.
- Some patients develop thrombocytopenia only, whereas others develop thrombosis.
- Few manifest devastating widespread thrombosis.
- Venous thrombosis is more common but can be arterial.
- Painful skin lesion at heparin injection sites.
- Occlusion of the distal extremities can lead to gangrene and require amputation.
- Diagnostic clue: Distal pulses are usually intact.
- Patients rarely have frank bleeding.

■ **Diagnosis**
- **HIT** is a clinical diagnosis.
- Abrupt decreases in platelet count by half.
- Platelet counts can be in the normal range, but the trend of decreasing by at least half is a useful diagnostic criterion.
- Patients have usually been exposed to heparin within the last 4 to 14 days.
- If HIT occurs during the first 3 days after heparin exposure, consider an amnestic response and search for prior heparin exposure.
- Heparin can be from any source; low-molecular-weight heparins, heparin, and any amount; heparin line flushes.
- HIT usually does not occur if the prior heparin exposure occurred more than 100 days earlier.
- Arterial or venous thrombosis can manifest.
- Heparin resistance: Patients requiring large doses of heparin to achieve a therapeutic activated partial thromboplastin time (aPTT).
- Enzyme-linked immunosorbent assay (ELISA) test is a helpful screening test to rule out HIT but can be overly sensitive.
- The serotonin release assay is more specific but is usually available only at specialized laboratories.
- Rely on clinical grounds for diagnosis.

■ **Treatment**
1. **Stop heparin:** all flushes, all sources.
2. Start a new agent: hirudin, danaparoid, argatroban, or other new agents.

3. Argatroban: direct thrombin inhibitor; cleared by the liver.
   2.0 µg/kg/min intravenously (IV) is the usual dose; 0.5 µg/kg/min if liver impairment.
   Warfarin and argatroban together prolong the international normalized ratio (INR) beyond that produced by warfarin alone.
   If the INR is more than 4.0, stop argatroban. Repeat the INR in 4 to 6 hours, and if in the therapeutic range, continue Coumadin. If below, resume argatroban and re-evaluate.
4. Danaparoid: heparinoid.
   Low *in vivo* cross-reactivity with HIT antibodies
5. Hirudin: direct thrombin inhibitor, renally cleared; bolus 0.4 mg/kg, infuse 0.15 mg/kg/hr, monitor aPTT to 1.5 to 2.5 times the normal, discontinue when INR is in the therapeutic range for 2 days.
6. Avoid giving Coumadin alone because of the possibility of a rapid drop in protein C, which could result in venous limb gangrene.
7. Do not use low-molecular-weight heparins because of their potential for cross-reactivity.
8. Treat until platelet count is normal.
   - Hidden sources of heparin: line flushes, catheters and guidewires, rinsing agents in surgical suite.
   - *Any* source of heparin, however small, can exacerbate HIT.

Idiopathic Thrombocytopenic Purpura

■ Epidemiology
- Common cause of thrombocytopenia in young adults, greater incidence in women

■ Etiology
- Idiopathic or primary ITP: adults, children, pregnant women
- Secondary: associated with lupus, rheumatoid arthritis, Crohn disease, primary biliary cirrhosis, lymphoproliferative disorders, viral hepatitis, HIV, after bone marrow transplantation, sarcoidosis, Evans syndrome, and possibly *Helicobacter pylori* infection

■ Pathophysiology
- IgG and immunoglobulin M (IgM) antibodies react with antigenic sites on platelets and cause platelet destruction by the mononuclear phagocytocytic system. The platelets are destroyed by the reticuloendothelial system in the liver and spleen.

■ Clinical Manifestations

- Patient presents with hemorrhagic manifestations: petechiae, purpura, epistaxis, menorrhagia, bleeding gums, or bleeding from any mucosal surface.
- Rarely GI tract bleeding or intracranial hemorrhage.
- The platelet count and pattern of bleeding do not always correlate.
- Wet purpura (mucosal bleeding) usually connotes a higher risk of serious bleeding.

■ Diagnosis

- Clinical diagnosis of exclusion, so always exclude medications and all other secondary causes.
- Platelet-associated antibodies are not helpful because of false-positive results.
- Platelet count can be very low; 3000 to 5000/liter.
- Platelet size and mean platelet volume (MPV) can be increased.
- Usually no splenomegaly, but if present, alternative diagnosis should be suspected.
- Bone marrow examination findings are normal and are not needed for the diagnosis. Some suggest if contemplating a splenectomy.
- Test for direct Coombs (DAT), if positive with concurrent ITP, diagnosis of Evans syndrome is made.
- Test for blood type if anti-D therapy is contemplated.

■ Treatment

- Treatment goals: Induce a long-term remission without ongoing medications.
- Complete correction of platelet count is *not* necessary.
- Treatment unnecessary if platelet count is more than $50,000 \times 10^6$ unless bleeding occurs.
- Before any treatment, immunize with pneumococcal, meningococcal, and *Haemophilus* vaccines in possible preparation for a splenectomy.
- First-line treatment: steroids, usually prednisone 1 mg/kg/day orally for 3 to 6 weeks; 70% will respond initially, but only 25% will respond long term. Alternative is dexamethasone (Decadron) 40 mg IV for 4 days, steroid pulse.
- Immediate treatment: Those at high risk, actively bleeding, or going for splenectomy have two options: intravenous immunoglobulin (IVIg) or intravenous anti-D.
- IVIg: 2 g/kg IV over 2 to 5 days depending on urgency. Should see effect in 48 to 72 hours; usually not durable; safe to use in pregnancy, but expensive. Side effects include allergic reactions,

volume overload, congestive heart failure, delayed renal toxicity, vascular thrombosis, and hyperviscosity.

- Anti-D: 75 µg/kg IV in one dose. Patient must be Rh D positive and have intact spleen. May have some activity in splenectomized patients because Kupffer cells in liver still present. General recommendation is to use other medications if no spleen. Be aware of hemoglobin drop and be careful in patients with positive DAT result. Should see effect in 48 to 72 hours, but not durable beyond a few weeks.
- Splenectomy: Approximately 60% achieve long-lasting remission after the spleen is removed. These patients are at risk for overwhelming postsplenectomy sepsis. Patients should carry a medical card/bracelet, have antibiotics at home, and take antimalarial prophylaxis if traveling to malarial areas.
- Other treatments: Recombinant factor 7a can be used in emergency situations with some benefit. Danazol, azathioprine, cyclophosphamide (either IV or orally), cyclosporine, pulse dexamethasone, rituxan, and vincristine have all been attempted with various success.

Drug Induced

- Heparin as mentioned previously.
- Quinidine, quinine, digoxin, valproic acid, cimetidine, chloramphenicol, penicillins, cocaine, chemotherapy drugs, and many others can cause thrombocytopenia.
- Ethanol causes selective megakaryocytic suppression.

Post-Transfusion Purpura

- One week after transfusion of any blood product.
- Rare, but bleeding can be life threatening.
- More commonly occurs in multiparous women.
- Antibody to the platelet antigen HPA-1a, which is lacking on the patients platelets.
- Patient usually sensitized from prior exposure to blood products or from prior pregnancy.
- Treatment: Only give HPA-1a–negative platelets. IVIg and steroids.

Autoimmune Disorders

- Evans syndrome: concurrent autoimmune hemolytic anemia and ITP; treat with steroids

- Concurrent autoimmune thyroid disorders: usually Graves disease or Hashimoto thyroiditis

Infection

- Septicemia, bacterial, viral, and fungal infections can lead to thrombocytopenia.
- HIV infection and hepatitis C can have an immunologic component to the thrombocytopenia.
- Usual treatment for all infectious causes of thrombocytopenia is to treat the underlying infection.

Disseminated Intravascular Coagulation

Increased thrombin generation, leading to a hemorrhagic process (usually in infections) or chronic thrombosis (usually in malignancy)

■ Associated Conditions

- Septicemia, obstetrical complications (amniotic fluid embolism, abruptio placentae, preeclampsia and eclampsia, septic abortion), intravascular hemolysis, leukemias (especially acute promyelocytic leukemia t[15;17]), solid malignancy, pancreatitis, burns, acute respiratory distress syndrome (ARDS), acidosis, crush injuries, severe trauma, cardiovascular disorders (aortic aneurysm, malignant hypertension, acute myocardial infarction, stroke, cardiac bypass surgery).

■ Pathophysiology

- Clotting proteins are activated to form excess thrombin by various stimuli, namely tissue factor. This may be initiated by head trauma or placental abruption, which both may release copious amounts of tissue factor into the circulation. Endothelial cell damage by endotoxin or cytokines may also trigger tissue factor. Procoagulants on malignant cells also activate tissue factor.
- Regardless of the initiator, the coagulation cascade is activated and at times overwhelmed; this leads to two possibilities:
  1. A chronic thrombotic process in which the coagulation proteins are compensated for by increased production
  2. An uncontrolled consumption of coagulation factors and platelets, leading to life-threatening bleeding
- Thrombotic complications are usually the result of cancer.
- Bleeding complications are acute and uncompensated and are triggered by the underlying event, usually septicemia.

■ Clinical Manifestations

- Bleeding (petechiae, purpura, oozing from intravenous sites)
- Fever, hypotension, acidosis, hypoxemia, and thrombosis

■ Laboratory Findings

- Schistocytes on peripheral smear
- Hypofibrinogenemia
- Prolonged prothrombin time
- Prolonged aPTT
- Prolonged thrombin time
- Thrombocytopenia
- Abnormal factor VIII
- Fibrin/fibrinogen degradation products
- D-Dimer elevation
- Fibrin monomer
- Prothrombin fragment 1+2
- Leukocytosis

■ Treatment (Table 8-1)

- Treat the initiating process.
- Decrease thrombin generation: Heparin, antithrombin concentrates, and activated protein C concentrates can be used.
- Blood product replacement: Platelets, cryoprecipitate to correct factor VIII and fibrinogen deficiencies, fresh frozen plasma to replace coagulation proteins, and packed RBCs to correct anemia.
- Antifibrinolytic agents are contraindicated in DIC.

Hemangiomas

- Kasabach-Merritt syndrome.
- Platelet consumption by localized intravascular coagulation within a congenital vascular tumor.
- A form of DIC.

■ TABLE 8-1 Disseminated Intravascular Coagulation Tests and Interventions

Tests	Intervention
International normalized ratio prolonged	Fresh frozen plasma until normal
Activated partial thromboplastin time prolonged	Fresh frozen plasma until normal
Fibrinogen low	Cryoprecipitate
Platelets low	Platelet count goal: >50,000/μl

- Treatment: surgical removal if possible.
- Most hemangiomas are not surgically removed and involute by adulthood.

Vascular Disease

- Congenital/acquired valvular disease
- Cardiopulmonary bypass surgery; most likely due to platelet aggregation and fragmentation in extracorporeal circulation
- Treatment: platelet transfusions

BONE MARROW FAILURE STATES

- Ethanol abuse: megakaryocytic suppression
- Nutritional deficiencies: megaloblastic anemia
- Marrow failure/infiltration: aplastic anemia, leukemia, tumor, metastatic cancer, multiple myeloma, myelofibrosis, and lymphoma
- Drugs: marrow suppression
- Inherited: rare and associated with other characteristic abnormalities; absent radii syndrome, Fanconi anemia, megakaryocytic hypoplasia

SEQUESTRATION

Hypersplenism

- Platelet sequestration due to splenomegaly (Box 8-2)
- Liver disease most common cause
- Liver spleen nuclear medicine scan helpful in diagnosis

■ BOX 8-2 Causes of Splenomegaly

- Infections: Epstein-Barr virus, cytomegalovirus, bacterial, protozoal
- Lymphoproliferative: myelofibrosis, chronic myeloid leukemia
- Leukemia: hairy cell leukemia
- Autoimmune: rheumatoid arthritis, systemic lupus erythematosus
- Storage disorders: Gaucher diseases
- Hemolysis: congenital: hereditary spherocytosis and acquired: autoimmune hemolysis
- Amyloid
- Portal vein thrombosis
- Metastatic cancer
- Liver disease: cirrhosis

DILUTIONAL

- Massive blood transfusion
- Plasma exchange

PREGNANCY

Incidental

- 10% drop in third trimester
- Mild thrombocytopenia, usually greater than 70,000
- Check for normal blood pressure to screen for preeclampsia

ITP of Pregnancy

- Diagnosis of exclusion.
- Treatment: IVIg; prednisone in low doses can be attempted.
- Route of delivery should be determined by maternal obstetrical indications.
- Routine caesarean section not shown to improve fetal outcome.
- Can be associated with fetal or neonatal thrombocytopenia.
- Only predictor of whether neonatal thrombocytopenia may be present is history of baby with thrombocytopenia.

Preeclampsia

- Hypertension, proteinuria, fluid retention, 30% have thrombocytopenia

HELLP Syndrome

- Hemolysis, elevated liver enzymes, low platelets, fragmented RBCs, high LDH
- Treatment for both: delivery

Acute Fatty Liver of Pregnancy

- Fulminant disorder in third trimester manifested by thrombocytopenia (platelet destruction), hypertension, proteinuria, impaired hepatic synthesis, and coagulopathy
- Treatment: urgent delivery

HEREDITARY THROMBOCYTOPENIA

- Rare disorders
- Wiskott-Aldrich syndrome: X linked, small platelets, associated with eczema, and increased susceptibility to infections
- May-Hegglin anomaly: autosomal dominant, huge platelets, Dohle bodies (inclusions in granulocytes)
- Bernard-Soulier syndrome: autosomal recessive, giant platelets, deficiency of the platelet glycoprotein Ib/V/IX complex, platelet aggregation is normal except for absent platelet agglutination with ristocetin

9 White Blood Cell Disorders

NEUTROPHILS

- Functions of the neutrophil include migrating to the sites of inflammation, phagocytosis, and destruction of invading microorganisms.
- Cytoplasm contains granules; nucleus has three to four segments.
- Life span is 1 to 2 days in tissues.
- Normal neutrophil count 4 to 10×10^9/L (depending on laboratory).

Neutrophilia

- Defined as an increase in the blood neutrophil count above 10×10^9/L
- Leukemoid reaction: a very high rise in white blood cell (WBC) count; usually mimics leukemia; caused by severe infection or malignancy
- Usually a reactive phenomenon; rarely a myeloproliferative process

■ Etiology

- Infection (bacterial, viral, fungal, any infectious process).
- Inflammation (trauma, infarction, stress, anxiety, epinephrine administration, rheumatoid disease, gout, vasculitis, colitis, nephritis, pancreatitis).
- Physical agents (cold, heat, burns, labor, surgery, anesthesia, pain, convulsions).
- Myeloproliferative disorders (chronic myeloid leukemia [CML], polycythemia vera [PV], essential thrombocythemia [ET], agnogenic myeloid metaplasia [AMM]): This is the main differentiation. Usually more than one cell line is affected, and the patient has splenomegaly or hepatomegaly.
- Cancer: Any tumor can cause a reactive neutrophilia.
- Tobacco use is probably the most common cause for a chronic low-grade neutrophilia.
- Postsplenectomy.
- Drugs: epinephrine, glucocorticoids, colony-stimulating factors, vaccines, venom, lithium, and other medications.

Neutropenia

- Defined as an absolute neutrophil count (ANC) less than 1800/μL.
- Percentage of segmented and banded neutrophils multiplied by total white blood cell (WBC) count equals the ANC.
- Mild neutropenia is an ANC between 1000 and 1800/μL.
- Moderate neutropenia is an ANC between 500 and 1000/μL.
- Severe neutropenia is an ANC between 0 and 500/μL.
- Neutrophil levels are lower in some racial groups: Africans, African Americans, and Jewish individuals.

■ Etiology

- Congenital: examples include Kostmann syndrome, cyclic neutropenia, Chédiak-Higashi syndrome, and others
- Drugs: anticonvulsants, antithyroids, phenothiazines, antiinflammatory, antibacterial, chemotherapy agents
- Autoimmune disorders: lupus, rheumatoid arthritis, Felty syndrome, splenomegaly, thyroiditis, idiopathic thrombocytopenia purpura (ITP), and autoimmune hemolytic anemia
- Large granular lymphocytosis
- Infection: human immunodeficiency virus (HIV), parvovirus, mononucleosis, sepsis, tuberculosis, typhoid
- Hematologic malignancies: acute myeloid leukemia (AML), myelodysplastic syndrome (MDS), chronic lymphocytic leukemia (CLL), lymphoma, thymoma, nutritional deficiencies

■ Infection Risk

- Highest risk at ANCs between 0 and 200/μL.
- Chronicity of the neutropenia places the patient at greater risk.

■ Symptoms

- Severe neutropenia: throat/mouth infections, oral ulceration, pharyngitis, skin infections, sinopulmonary infections, septicemia, fever, mucosal abscesses

■ Workup

- If evidence of a fever >100.5°F (38.1°C), the patient should be pan-cultured.

■ Treatment

- Neutropenia is considered a medical emergency.
- Begin aggressive evaluation and early institution of broad-spectrum antibiotics immediately.

- Avoid rectal or vaginal examination in a neutropenic patient because spontaneous bacteremia can occur with enteric/vaginal organisms.

LYMPHOCYTES

- Two principle types: B and T cells
- B cells: humoral immunity via antibody secretion
- T cells: cell-mediated immunity

Lymphocytosis

- Peripheral blood lymphocyte counts more than 4.5×10^9/L

■ Etiology
- Leukemias and lymphomas: CLL, acute lymphocytic leukemia, non-Hodgkin lymphoma, Hodgkin disease, hairy cell leukemia, Waldenström macroglobulinemia, adult T-cell leukemia/lymphoma, large granular lymphocytosis
- Infections: Epstein-Barr virus (infectious mononucleosis), cytomegalovirus, mumps, varicella, hepatitis, adenovirus, influenza, virtually any viral infection
- Trauma
- Stress: myocardial infarction, sickle crisis, burns, uremia
- Rheumatoid disease
- Epinephrine
- Exercise
- Postsplenectomy

Lymphopenia

■ Etiology
- Hematologic diseases: MDS, Hodgkin disease, angioimmunoblastic lymphadenopathy
- Infections: acquired immunodeficiency syndrome
- Collagen vascular disease
- Drugs: chemotherapy
- Trauma: surgery, burns
- Renal failure
- Liver failure
- Anorexia nervosa
- Aplastic anemia
- Cushing disease

- Sarcoidosis
- Rare congenital disorders

MONOCYTES

- Monocytes are part of the reticuloendothelial system and become macrophages in the tissues.
- Lung alveolar macrophages, Kupffer cells in the liver, histiocytes, macrophages in lymph nodes, spleen, and liver.

Monocytosis

- Peripheral blood monocyte counts greater than $0.8 \times 10^9/L$

■ Etiology

- Inflammatory conditions: sarcoidosis, lupus.
- Infections: malaria, trypanosomiasis, typhoid, tuberculosis, infective endocarditis, syphilis, brucellosis.
- Hematologic malignancies: MDS, Hodgkin disease, AML (subtype M4 or M5), chronic myelomonocytic leukemia.
- After chemotherapy: Monocytes are the first cell to increase after aplasia.

Monocytopenia

- Peripheral blood less than $0.2 \times 10^9/L$

■ Etiology

- Hairy cell leukemia, MDS, aplastic anemia
- Drugs: glucocorticoids, chemotherapy
- Autoimmune disorders
- Cyclic neutropenia
- Thermal injuries

BASOPHILS

- Basophils form mast cells in tissues.
- Degranulation of these cells results in hypersensitivity reactions.
- Basophils have a short life span of 1 to 2 days.

Basophilia

- Peripheral blood basophil count greater than $0.1 \times 10^9/L$

■ **Etiology**

- Myeloproliferative disorders: CML, PV, ET, AMM, basophilic leukemia
- Hypothyroidism
- Recovery from infection
- Inflammatory disorders, rheumatoid diseases, ulcerative colitis
- Drugs: estrogens
- Viral infections
- Irradiation
- Hyperlipidemia

Basopenia

- Peripheral blood basophil counts less than 0.1×10^9/L

■ **Etiology**

- Acute rheumatic fever
- Stress
- Thyrotoxicosis
- Lobar pneumonia
- After steroid therapy
- Cushing syndrome
- Drugs: progesterones
- Bleeding
- Allergic reactions

EOSINOPHILS

Eosinophilia

- Peripheral blood eosinophilia more than 0.7×10^9/L

■ **Etiology**

- Drugs
- Parasitic infections: hookworm, *Ascaris*, tapeworms, filariasis, schistosomiasis, amoebiasis
- Allergies: asthma, eczema, urticaria
- Skin disease: pemphigus, dermatitis herpetiformis
- Malignancy: Hodgkin disease
- Polyarteritis nodosa, sarcoid
- Irradiation
- Hypereosinophilic syndromes: history of allergy, cough, fever, and pulmonary infiltrates on chest x-ray

- Eosinophilic leukemia
- AML with eosinophils
- T-cell lymphomas

Eosinophilopenia

■ **Etiology**

- After steroids
- After stress
- Cushing syndrome

10 Bleeding Disorders

Inherited Disorders of the Coagulation System

■ Hemophilia A

Hemophilia A is caused by a deficiency in *factor VIII*.

- The genetic defect occurs on the X chromosome, and about half of the mutations are novel somatic mutations, so affected boys may not reveal a family history of bleeding.
- The disorder affects about 1 in 10,000 people.
- Laboratory studies reveal a prolonged activated partial thromboplastin time (aPTT).
- The treatment for active bleeding is transfusion of cryoprecipitate or factor VIII itself.
- Clinical manifestations are listed in Table 10-1.

■ Hemophilia B

Hemophilia B is also known as Christmas disease; these patients are deficient in *factor IX*.

- This disorder is much less common, affecting only 1 in 100,000 people.
- The clinical manifestations are similar to those listed in Table 10-1.
- The treatment for active bleeding is fresh frozen plasma (FFP) or factor IX.

■ Factor XI Deficiency

- Autosomal recessive inheritance, especially in Ashkenazi Jews
- Variable bleeding patterns, usually only after trauma or postoperatively
- No clear relationship between the amount deficient and degree of bleeding
- Treat by replacing with FFP

■ Factor XII Deficiency

- Patients with factor XII deficiency can have significant prolongation of the partial thromboplastin time (PTT), but without clinically significant bleeding.
- They can go to surgery without special interventions to normalize the PTT.

■ TABLE 10-1 Clinical Manifestations of Hemophilia A

Clinical Severity	Amount of Factor VIII Present	Manifestations
Mild hemophilia	>5%	May bleed after trauma or surgery
Moderate hemophilia	2% to 5%	Usually only bleed after trauma or surgery
Severe hemophilia	<2%	Spontaneous bleeds into muscles and joints

■ TABLE 10-2 Classification of von Willebrand Disease

Type I	Partial deficit of vWF	Autosomal dominant inheritance
Type II	Qualitative defect of vWf	Autosomal dominant inheritance
Type III	Complete deficiency (rare)	Autosomal recessive inheritance

■ Von Willebrand Disease

Von Willebrand disease is a primary platelet disorder characterized by a deficiency in von Willebrand factor (vWf).

- vWf sits on the endothelial surface and binds **platelet glycoprotein Ib/IX**, thus initiating platelet adhesion and activation.
- The incidence is as high as 1%.
- Men and women are affected equally.
- There are three types (Table 10-2).
- Most patients with clinically significant von Willebrand disease
will give a positive family history of bleeding (e.g., postsurgical
and menorrhagia) and a personal history of easy bruising and/or
mucosal bleeding.
- Laboratory evaluation reveals a prolonged bleeding time and a
prolonged aPTT in more than half of patients.
- Treatment usually involves **desmopressin (DDAVP)**, a vaso-
pressin analogue that stimulates release of endogenous vWf.
  - Works in type I and variably in type II.
  - Does not work in type III.
  - Cannot use for longer than 48 hours, because the body's
  vWf stores become depleted.
- Plasma vWf levels are reduced in patients with type O blood and
during pregnancy, but this is not usually clinically significant.

■ Glanzmann Thrombasthenia

Glanzmann thrombasthenia is an autosomal recessive deficiency
of platelet glycoprotein IIb/IIIa, which is important in platelet
aggregation.

■ Bernard-Soulier Syndrome

Bernard-Soulier syndrome is an autosomal recessive deficiency of platelet glycoprotein 1b/IX, which is necessary for platelet adhesion to the endothelium.

■ Gray Platelet Syndrome

Gray platelet syndrome is a platelet granule deficiency that results in a weak platelet activation response.

■ Afibrinogenemia

Afibrinogenemia usually manifests as postoperative bleeding; there are also some inherited disorders of fibrinogen function (dysfibrinogenemias).

Acquired Disorders of the Coagulation System

■ Acquired Hemophilia

- Rare, with only 1 in 1,000,000 per year
- The etiology is usually anti-factor VIII autoantibodies, although other anti-factor antibodies are seen as well.
- 40% of cases are associated with other conditions including the following:
  - Pregnancy (usually postpartum 1 to 4 mo, up to 1 yr)
  - Autoimmune diseases, especially lupus, rheumatoid arthritis, graft-versus-host disease
  - Underlying malignancies (in 10%), especially lymphoproliferative disorders
  - Drugs, especially penicillin, sulfas, anticonvulsants
- Patients may present with spontaneous hematomas, hemorrhage into muscle or skin, or prolonged postoperative or postpartum bleeding that is severe and difficult to control.
- Laboratory evaluation reveals a prolonged aPTT, which does not correct with 50/50 mixing study (i.e., patient's serum mixed with equal parts normal serum).
- The central tenets of treatment are (1) to stop the bleeding and then (2) to destroy the inhibitor.
- DDAVP can be effective in patients with low antibody titers, although factor replacement is necessary when the titers are high.
- Plasmapheresis can be performed if bleeding is significant.
- Prednisone plus cyclophosphamide and sometimes intravenous immunoglobulin have been the mainstay of immunosuppressive therapy; rituxan appears to be effective as well.

■ Medication Related

Medication-related bleeding must be ruled out; ask about use of aspirin, nonsteroidal antiinflammatory drugs, clopidogrel, ticlopid, Coumadin, and heparin.

■ Uremia

Uremia prolongs bleeding time either because of uremia itself or because of a toxic inhibitor that is a byproduct of the elevated blood urea nitrogen level.

■ Post–Coronary Artery Bypass Graft

Platelet counts may be within the normal range in post–coronary artery bypass graft, but they are degranulated secondary to activation by the bypass machine, and thus, they are ineffective.

■ Paraproteins

For example, multiple myeloma and monoclonal gammopathy of undetermined significance (MGUS); globulin fraction (total protein–albumin) must be greater than 6 g to inhibit platelets.

■ Liver Dysfunction

Liver dysfunction is usually due to a combination of decreased clotting factors and splenomegaly.

■ Vitamin K Deficiency

Vitamin K deficiency is due to decreased intake in the poor or elderly or decreased absorption as in postsurgical patients.

■ Dysfibrinogenemia

Dysfibrinogenemia can occur in liver disease, acquired immunodeficiency syndrome, and lymphoproliferative disorders.

Thrombosis

THROMBOSIS

■ Epidemiology

- Deep venous thrombosis (DVT) is a common disease, with an annual incidence of 1 per 1000.
- 200,000 cases are diagnosed per year in the United States.
- 20% die suddenly of pulmonary embolism (PE).
- DVT and PE usually coexist.

■ Pathogenesis

- **Virchow triad**: venous stasis, vessel wall injury, and hypercoagulable state

■ Risk Factors

- Arterial thrombosis is secondary to smoking, hypertension, hyperlipidemia, and diabetes mellitus.
- Up to 40% of people develop DVT after orthopedic or major abdominal surgery, as well as one third of medical patients and patients in the intensive care unit.
- Cancer is a thrombotic risk factor, as exemplified by Trousseau syndrome (migratory thrombophlebitis in the setting of a malignancy), which may be occult or predate the diagnosis. Cancer types that are most often correlated with thrombotic events are brain, ovarian, pancreatic, lung, and colon.
- Inflammatory disorders, hemolytic anemias, myeloproliferative disorders, and hormonal pills (estrogen, oral contraceptive pills [OCPs], tamoxifen) predispose to thrombosis.

■ Etiology

- **Thrombophilia** is an inherited or acquired disorder of the hemostatic mechanism predisposing to thrombosis, which may be arterial or venous. Inherited and acquired types are divided and discussed in detail.

INHERITED THROMBOPHILIA

■ Epidemiology

Estimated frequency is as follows:
- Antithrombin (AT) deficiency: 1%
- Protein C deficiency: 5%
- Protein S deficiency: 3%
- Factor V Leiden mutation: 20%
- Prothrombin 20210 deficiency: 6%

■ Pathogenesis

Tendency toward venous thrombosis arising from the following:
1. Hyperactive coagulation pathway proteins
2. Hypoactive anticoagulation pathways
3. Hypoactive fibrinolysis

■ Risk Factors

- Most people will never develop a thrombosis.
- A threshold effect is usually needed, such as a thrombotic predisposition and pregnancy or a long plane ride.
- The example is below
- Factor V Leiden mutation and OCPs have a synergistically increased clotting risk versus that of either alone.

■ Clinical Manifestations

- Venous thrombosis (>90% of the cases)
- DVT (lower limbs is the most common site of thrombosis)
- PE (risk of PE is highest in an iliofemoral clot > femoral > popliteal > calf vein thrombosis)
- Superficial thrombophlebitis
- Mesenteric vein thrombosis, cerebral vein thrombosis (rare but characteristic)
- Family history of thrombosis
- First thrombosis at young age (<45 years)
- Frequent recurrences

■ Etiology

- AT deficiency
- Protein C deficiency
- Protein S deficiency
- Factor V Leiden mutation
- Prothrombin 20210 mutation

Antithrombin Deficiency

■ Epidemiology
- Autosomal dominant; 1 in 600 people have AT deficiency.
- Median age at first thrombosis is 24 years.
- AT used to be classified as AT-III, which is now considered old nomenclature.

■ Pathogenesis
- AT is synthesized in the liver and endothelial cells.
- AT acts as an anticoagulant by directly binding and inactivating serine proteases in the clotting cascade: thrombin, Xa, IXa, and XIa.
- The presence of heparin increases the activity of AT by more than 1000-fold.

■ Clinical Manifestations
- Resistance to heparin, thus requiring high doses.
- Thrombosis risk increases during pregnancy.
- Risk for thrombosis is higher than for protein C, protein S, or factor V Leiden mutation.

■ Diagnosis
- Functional assay is the initial screen.
- Heparin will decrease AT levels; OCPs and Coumadin will increase levels.
- Acquired conditions must be ruled out, including nephrotic syndrome, liver disease, disseminated intravascular coagulation (DIC), preeclampsia, asparaginase, and chemotherapy.

Protein C and S Deficiency

■ Epidemiology
- Autosomal dominant.
- Heterozygotes: Risk of thrombosis is sevenfold; 1 in 300 people have deficiencies of protein C or S.
- Homozygotes: neonatal purpura fulminans; usually fatal.
- Median age at first clot is 24 years.

■ Pathogenesis
- Vitamin K–dependent plasma proteins synthesized in the liver.
- Protein S acts as a cofactor for protein C; 60% of protein S is bound to C4b binding protein.
- C4b is an acute-phase reactant and can lower free protein S in inflammatory and related conditions.

■ Clinical Manifestations

- Warfarin-induced skin necrosis: Seen in heterozygotes; skin necrosis from rapid reduction in already low protein C levels.
- Suspect diagnosis in patients with painful red skin lesions developing a few days after starting Coumadin.
- Arterial thrombosis is seen in patients with protein S deficiency.

■ Diagnosis

- Coumadin will decrease levels.
- Acute thrombosis will alter levels; not the ideal time for testing.
- Check erythrocyte sedimentation rate (ESR) and C-reactive protein (CRP) concurrent with protein S levels.
- Rule out acquired conditions, including nephrotic syndrome, liver disease, DIC, preeclampsia, asparaginase use, and chemotherapy.

Activated Protein C Resistance

■ Etiology

- 95% of the time caused by factor V Leiden mutation
- Other causes: OCPs, rare genetic defects in factor V and VIII, or lupus anticoagulant

Factor V Leiden Mutation

■ Epidemiology

- Autosomal dominant; 3% to 8% of whites are heterozygotes for factor V Leiden mutation and 1 in 1000 are homozygotes.
- Heterozygotes have an eightfold increase in thrombotic relative risk.
- Homozygotes have a 91-fold increased risk of thrombotic events.

■ Pathogenesis

- Point mutation in factor V; glutamine to arginine at amino acid 506 in 95% of cases.
- This mutation renders the factor V molecule resistant to cleavage by activated protein C (APC).
- Thrombosis occurs because the altered factor Va still has the same procoagulant activity as normal factor Va.

■ Risk Factors

- OCP use multiplies the risk: 28-fold increased thrombotic risk for heterozygotes, 270-fold increased thrombotic risk for homozygotes.

■ **Diagnosis**

- DNA diagnostic methods allow testing at any time.
- Coumadin and heparin have no effect on testing.

Prothrombin 20210 Mutation

■ **Epidemiology**

- Found in 2% to 3% of whites

■ **Pathogenesis**

- G to A substitution in the 3′ untranslated region of the pro-thrombin gene.
- Mutation associated with elevated levels of the prothrombin molecule.
- Patients with increased concentrations of prothrombin also have an increased risk of thrombosis.

■ **Diagnosis**

- DNA diagnostic methods allow testing at any time.
- Coumadin and heparin have no effect on testing.

Elevated Factor VIII

■ **Epidemiology**

- Not known at this time

■ **Pathogenesis**

- The specific genetic defect or polymorphism has not been detected yet.

■ **Risk Factors**

- Associated fivefold increased risk of thrombosis

■ **Diagnosis**

- More than 150% factor VIII level as measured by an activity assay confers the thrombotic risk.
- Elevated factor VIII levels can be associated with inflammatory states: infection, inflammatory bowel disease, group O blood type, and increased von Willebrand factor.
- Rule out acquired causes with ESR or CRP testing along with factor VIII levels.
- Suspect in patients with shortened activated partial thrombo-plastin time (aPTT).
- Repeat in 6 weeks with ESR.

■ BOX 11-1 Acquired Thrombotic Disorders

- Antiphospholipid disorders: lupus anticoagulant, anticardiolipin antibodies
- Hyperhomocysteinemia
- Cancer: during chemotherapy
- Surgery: orthopedic, abdominal, and cancer operations
- Trauma: hip fracture, acute spinal injury
- Sedentary
- Obesity
- Tobacco usage
- Hospital admission: major medical illnesses (acute respiratory failure, pneumonia, acute myocardial infarction, congestive heart failure, ischemic stroke)
- Myeloproliferative disorders
- Paroxysmal nocturnal hemoglobinuria
- Autoimmune disorders
- Inflammatory disorders: inflammatory bowel disease
- Hemolytic anemias
- Nephrosis
- Estrogens, oral contraceptive pills
- Hyperlipidemia: elevated lipoprotein (a)
- Pregnancy and puerperium
- Heparin induced thrombocytopenia
- Disseminated intravascular coagulation
- Thrombotic purpura

ACQUIRED THROMBOTIC DISORDERS

- Common acquired thrombotic disorders are outlined in Box 11-1.
- The most common are discussed in more detail in the following sections.

Antiphospholipid Disorders

■ Epidemiology

- Antiphospholipid disorders occur in 2% of the population.

■ Pathogenesis

- **Lupus anticoagulant** (LA) is a paradoxical name for a common clotting disorder.
- Immunoglobulin G/immunoglobulin M autoantibodies that cause prolongation of phospholipid-dependent coagulation tests.
- Autoantibodies directed against cell surface glycoproteins in concert with anionic phospholipids. B2-glycoprotein-a, prothrombin, and Immunoglobulin A are the most notable proteins.

- Anticardiolipin antibodies (ACAs) directed against proteins: B2-glycoprotein-1 or prothrombin, detected by solid-phase assays; enzyme-linked immunosorbent assay (ELISA).
- The mechanism of thrombosis is not known.

■ Clinical Manifestations

- LA and ACAs are associated with venous and arterial thrombosis, fetal loss, migraine, thrombocytopenia, livedo reticularis, heart valve disease, myelopathy, and devastating widespread thrombotic syndrome.
- Can be associated with bleeding by causing hypoprothrombinemia.
- Associated with autoimmune disorders, lymphoproliferative disorders, human immunodeficiency virus, drug reactions, and infections.

■ Diagnosis

Lupus Anticoagulant Tests

- Prolongs any phospholipid-dependent coagulation test: aPTT, Russell viper venom time, dilute prothrombin time.
- Does not correct with mixing study, inferring inhibitor.
- Inhibitory activity neutralized by adding excess phospholipid.
- Exclude factor VIII inhibitor.

Anticardiolipin Tests

- Detected by solid-phase assays: ELISA.

■ Treatment

- If there is no history of thrombosis, no treatment is needed. Careful follow-up is suggested.
- Patients with a thrombotic event should be treated indefinitely because the risk of recurrent thrombosis is high.
- International normalized ratio (INR) of 2.5 to 3.5 is recommended if an arterial event.
- Recurrent abortion: aspirin and low-molecular-weight heparins (LMWHs).
- Surgery prophylaxis: History of thrombosis should receive LMWHs.

Hyperhomocysteinemia

■ Epidemiology

- Most common form: Mutation at nucleotide 677 (GtoT) in the methylene tetrahydrofolate reductase enzyme causes loss of enzymatic activity.

- Rare severe homozygous form is called congenital homocystinuria: neurologic defects, premature atherosclerosis, thromboembolic disease, and mental retardation.

■ Pathogenesis

- Mechanism of action for thrombosis is not known.

■ Differential Diagnosis

- Deficiencies in folate, B_{12}, or B_6, renal disease, lupus, and tobacco use can all lead to elevated homocysteine levels.

■ Clinical Manifestations

- Mild hyperhomocysteinemia can cause arterial and venous thrombosis.

■ Treatment

- Folic acid replacement, sometimes with doses up to 5 mg/day.
- Vitamins B_6 and B_{12} replacement.
- Never begin folic acid without first checking for B_{12} deficiency by measuring serum methylmalonic acid (more sensitive test) and B_{12} levels.

Diagnostic Evaluation of Deep Venous Thrombosis

- DVT can be diagnosed by duplex ultrasound (sensitivity and specificity are 95% in symptomatic proximal DVT), contrast venography, magnetic resonance venography, impedance plethysmography, and venous phase helical computed tomography.
- The challenge of diagnosis lies in distinguishing acute from chronic DVT. Reimaging after 6 months can be useful to establish a new baseline comparison if a new clot develops in the same area.
- PE: Ventilation-perfusion scan (high probability scan suggests likelihood of PE in the range of 80%), helical spiral computed tomography (helpful if other lung processes occurring at same time and to view lung parenchyma), magnetic resonance angiography, pulmonary angiography (gold standard, invasive).
- Venous thrombotic workup involves ruling out obvious risk factors.
- If a clinician is unable to find an obvious risk factor or the suspicion is high for an inherited or acquired thrombotic disorder, a clotting panel should be obtained. Tests for venous and arterial thrombotic events are outlined in Boxes 11-2 and 11-3, respectively.

■ BOX 11-2 Venous Thrombotic Workup

- Rule out obvious causes
- Activated protein C resistance*
- Lupus anticoagulant*
- Anticardiolipin antibodies by enzyme-linked immunosorbent assay
- Prothrombin 20210 mutation testing by polymerase chain reaction
- Antithrombin activity (functional)*
- Protein C and S activity (functional)*
- Factor VIII level with sedimentation rate or C-reactive protein
- Fasting total plasma homocysteine level
- Factor V Leiden mutation
- D-Dimer
- Complete blood cell count

Older than 55 years, no other cause found, computed tomography scan of chest/abdomen/pelvis screen for cancer.
*Preferable to not test in the setting of acute clot or heparin or Coumadin treatment.

■ BOX 11-3 Arterial Thrombotic Workup

- Venous workup
- Transthoracic echocardiogram with bubble study looking for patent shunt, foramen ovale
- Lipid panel and lipoprotein (a)

Treatment of Venous Thrombosis/Pulmonary Embolism

- Acute management is with heparin or an LMWH.
- The goal is to rapidly reduce thrombin generation, prevent thrombus extension, and serve as a bridge to an oral anticoagulant.
- LMWHs are superior to heparin in most studies. LMWHs have a longer plasma half-life, better bioavailability, and more predictable pharmakinetics, and they may be given once or twice a day, are available as outpatient treatment, and have a lower incidence of heparin-induced thrombocytopenia than heparin.
- LMWHs need monitoring only in renal disease and extreme obesity; can be accomplished by sending an anti-Xa assay.
- Oral anticoagulants are started after heparin or LMWH and continued for up to 6 months. Experts advise continuing LMWH for 2 more days once the INR is therapeutic.

- Chronic anticoagulation is given for certain thrombotic disorders; assess each individual risk.
- Venal caval filters are best avoided if possible. Even though they protect against PE acutely, there is an increased risk of DVT after a filter is placed. Thus, the patient ideally will still need oral anticoagulation long term. Vena caval filters should be used only in patients who cannot be treated with anticoagulants because of contraindicatory bleeding or a very high likelihood of future bleeding.
- Thrombolytic therapy in the form of recombinant tissue plasminogen activator (TPA) should be given in patients with PE and cardiovascular collapse or compromise. Thrombolytic therapy in other situations requires much more investigation.
- TPA works well only in the acute setting.
- Postphlebitic syndrome (mild edema to severe limb swelling with pain and ulceration) can be prevented by treating a

---

■ TABLE 11-1 General Guidelines for Duration of Treatment Time for Anticoagulation

Condition	Duration
Provoked DVT	3 to 6 mo
Idiopathic DVT	6 mo
Idiopathic DVT, recurrent	Indefinite
Cancer	Until cancer is no longer active
Idiopathic PE	Indefinite
ITD and no history of clotting	No treatment
DVT and antiphospholipid syndrome	Indefinite
Recurrent DVT and ITD	Indefinite

DVT, deep venous thrombosis; ITD, inherited thrombotic disorder; PE, pulmonary embolism.

■ BOX 11-4 Patients Who Are at *High* Risk for Thrombosis Recurrence after the Standard 6 Months of Anticoagulation

- Active cancer or receiving chemotherapy
- Hyperhomocysteinemia
- Antiphospholipid antibodies
- Antithrombin, protein C or S deficiency
- Homozygous factor V Leiden mutation, not heterozygous
- Inflammatory bowel disease
- Multiple minor risk factors
- Recurrent idiopathic thrombosis

Current recommendation is to continue anticoagulants indefinitely, unless risk of bleeding is high in a specific individual situation.

thrombotic event in a timely manner. Providing adequate and aggressive anticoagulation, prescribing compressive stockings, and elevating the leg when possible help prevent postphlebitic syndrome. Iliofemoral thrombosis may benefit from thrombolytic therapy.

- General guidelines for duration of anticoagulant treatment are given in Table 11-1.
- Provoked DVT is defined as thrombosis with an obvious cause, such as a long plane trip, cancer, or after surgery.
- Patients who are at high risk of thrombotic recurrence are listed in Box 11-4. Current recommendation for the high-risk individuals is to continue anticoagulants indefinitely, unless risk of bleeding is high in a specific individual situation.

Hemochromatosis

Hemochromatosis

- Hemochromatosis is a genetic defect that leads to increased absorption of dietary iron.

■ Epidemiology

- Inherited autosomal recessive in 1% of population.
- 10% to 14% of whites of northern European descent are heterozygotes for the most common mutation.
- 1 in 250 are homozygotes for the condition.
- Hereditary hemochromatosis is rare in African Americans or Asians.

■ Genetics

- HFE gene was cloned in 1996 and localized to chromosome 6.
- The HFE protein is thought to be a key regulator in the active absorption of iron.
- Two mutations in the HFE gene have been found to account for most cases of hereditary hemochromatosis.
- The first mutation is a G-to-A substitution at nucleotide 845, leading to a cysteine-to-tyrosine substitution at amino acid position 282, called C282Y.
- The second mutation is a G-to-C substitution at nucleotide position 187, leading to a histidine-to-aspartic acid substitution at amino acid position 63, called H63D.
- C282Y/C282Y, homozygotes for the HFE gene, will develop hemochromatosis.
- C282Y/wild type(WT): Patients develop hemochromatosis only with another concurrent risk factor, such as alcohol consumption.
- H63D/H63D, homozygotes: only a small minority of these individuals will develop hemochromatosis.
- C282Y/H63D, compound heterozygotes, mild iron overload, evaluate for other risk factors.
- H63D/WT: rarely develop hemochromatosis without other risk factors.

■ Pathophysiology

- Iron overload.
- Absence in humans of a physiological mechanism to excrete excess iron.
- Continual iron intake (dietary or transfusional in the form of red blood cells) can result in iron overload and tissue damage, especially in the liver, heart, and pancreas, but can affect any organ.
- Failure to regulate iron absorption from bowel causing progressive increase in total body iron levels.
- Accumulation of iron starts first in the liver, then in the pancreas, heart, skin, and other organs.
- Once approximately 10 to 15 g of iron overload has occurred, symptoms begin.
- Alcohol consumption can advance time to symptoms as a second comorbidity.
- HFE gene is the primary protein thought to regulate iron absorption at the level of the enterocyte. Many other proteins are involved in the complicated process of iron transport and storage.

■ Clinical Manifestations

HEPATIC Mnemonic

- **H**epatic manifestations: hepatomegaly, chronic hepatitis, fibrosis, cirrhosis, hepatocellular carcinoma
- **E**ndocrine dysfunction: diabetes, hypothyroidism, hypoparathyroidism, adrenal insufficiency
- **P**ain: abdominal, unknown etiology in 25% of patients
- **A**rthritis: chondrocalcinosis
- **T**ransferrin saturation: most reliable indicator of iron overload
- **I**mpotence: gonadal dysfunction and hypogonadism
- **C**ardiac dysfunction: cardiomyopathy, heart failure, dysrhythmias

Other Symptoms

- Skin changes: pigmentation; slate gray or bronze discoloration; "bronze diabetes" term used to describe color discoloration with concurrent diabetes; usually a late finding.
- Fatigue: usually the first symptom
- Amenorrhea, loss of libido
- Depression, weight loss
- Body hair loss

Diagnostic Evaluation

- High index of suspicion is required.
- Liver biopsy used to be the sine qua non of the diagnosis of hemochromatosis; now rarely done and not needed.

- Diagnosis usually suspected when iron panel obtained for some other reason or liver function test abnormality.

Laboratory Tests
- Liver function tests.
- Serum iron can be elevated.
- Percentage of transferrin saturation more than 45% in women and more than 60% in men suggests hemochromatosis; elevated very early in disease; recommended as the most reliable indicator if iron overload.
- Serum ferritin: There is some correlation with iron stores but can be elevated as acute-phase reactant. Very high levels can be seen in acute hepatic necrosis.
- Differential: Aplastic anemia or ineffective erythropoiesis can cause high serum iron level, elevated percentage saturation, and high ferritin levels.
- Genetic testing: missense mutation on chromosome 6, a single point mutation, either C282Y or H63D.
- Annual liver ultrasound and serum α-fetoprotein performed to screen for hepatocellular carcinoma.
- Iron overload in African Americans still requires a liver biopsy. Genetic tests performed, but a normal genetic test result should not deter a liver biopsy.

■ Treatment
- Encourage patient to avoid alcohol, medicinal iron, ascorbic acid, iron skillets, and raw seafood. Raw seafood causes susceptibility to certain infections.
- Phlebotomy removes 450 mL of blood, which is approximately 250 mg of iron.
- Generally phlebotomy is performed every week and then on a maintenance schedule.
- Goals of phlebotomy: iron exhaustion, ferritin less than 20 µg/L, transferrin saturation less than 10%. Decreased mean corpuscular volume will be the first sign of iron exhaustion.

■ Prognosis
- Patients who do not have cirrhosis have a normal life span.
- Patients with cirrhosis who are treated promptly have a slightly compromised life span.
- Patients who present with advanced cirrhosis, ascites, and cardiac failure have a very poor prognosis.
- Patients who develop cirrhosis have a more than 200-fold increased risk of hepatocellular carcinoma.

Secondary Hemochromatosis

- Usually seen more in a hematologic disorder that necessitates frequent blood transfusions; for example, thalassemia major, X-linked sideroblastic anemia, sickle cell anemia, myelodysplasia.
- Also called transfusional hemosiderosis.
- Phlebotomy usually not an option because the patients is already anemic from his or her primary disorder.
- Iron is removed by chelating agents, most commonly deferoxamine.
- Deferoxamine is given intravenously over many hours, many times necessitating an indwelling pump that the patient wears at nighttime.
- Deferoxamine can cause ocular and auditory complications.

13 Transfusion Medicine

BLOOD PRODUCTS

Whole Blood

- 450 mL contains all the cells, plasma, and proteins.
- Little indication for use except in massive bleeding, such as trauma.

■ Packed Red Blood Cells

- Derived from whole blood; plasma removed sterilely.
- Components still in blood include the following:
  1. Packed red blood cells (RBCs)
  2. Solution to make less viscous, for example, acid citrate dextrose, adenosine saline solution
  3. Scant white blood cells (WBCs)
  4. Scant platelets
  5. Antibodies to non-native RBCs: for example, type B blood has circulating anti-A antibodies
  6. Cytokines produced by WBCs
  7. Small amount of plasma
- Can store for up to 42 days
- Volume approximately 240 mL
- One unit of packed RBCs expected to raise hemoglobin by 1 g/dL.
- Tracking hemoglobin values after transfusion, a directly measured value, more accurate than following hematocrit values

■ Leukocyte-Depleted Red Blood Cells

- Blood passed through a filter to remove 99% of the leukocytes.
- Lose 20% of the RBCs. Usually filtered before storage.
- Decreased risk of febrile nonhemolytic transfusion reactions; induced by leukocyte-derived cytokines.
- Decreased risk of cytomegalovirus (CMV) transmission.
- Decreased risk of alloimmunization to human leukocyte antigen (HLA) on WBCs. This prevents future platelet refractoriness.

■ CMV-Negative Red Blood Cells

- Used in transfusing CMV-negative patients who are immunocompromised or CMV-negative bone marrow transplant recipients.

■ Irradiated Red Blood Cells

- Blood irradiated with a minimum of 25 Gy to destroy donor T cells
- Indicated to stop transfusion-associated graft-versus-host disease: graft attacking host
- Useful in the following indications:
  1. After total body irradiation or bone marrow transplant
  2. Patients treated with purine analogues (fludarabine)
  3. Immunodeficient individuals
  4. Patients taking any immunosuppressive medication for any reason
  5. Transfusion from first-degree relative
  6. Patients with chronic lymphocytic leukemia
  7. Patients with hematologic malignancies: lymphoma, Hodgkin disease, acute myeloid leukemia (AML), acute lymphocytic leukemia (ALL)
  8. HLA-matched and/or cross-matched platelets

■ Washed Red Blood Cells

- Suspended in saline washes, must use in 24 hours
- Removes 85% of leukocytes, 99% of plasma, removes plasma proteins that cause allergic reactions
- Useful in immunoglobulin M (IgM) cold antibody hemolytic anemia
- Useful in immunoglobulin A (IgA)–deficient patients
- Useful in patients with allergic reactions
- Useful in patients with paroxysmal nocturnal hemoglobinuria (PNH)

■ Frozen Red Blood Cells

- Useful for prolonged RBC storage; rare blood cell types
- Same qualities as washed RBCs

ABO Compatibility

- Determining the ABO typing is the most important blood serology test (Tables 13-1 and 13-2).
- Group A specificity confers an RBC with galactosamine on the RBC. Type A persons have antibodies to type B blood. Can receive type A or O blood.

■ TABLE 13-1 Frequency of Blood Types in the United States

Type	Frequency
O+	38.0%
A+	36.0%
B+	8.0%
O−	7.0%
A−	6.0%
AB+	3.4%
B−	1.5%
AB−	0.6%

■ TABLE 13-2 Blood Product Compatibility

Type of Blood	Required Component Type
Whole blood	Must be identical to recipient's
RBCs	Must be compatible with recipient's plasma
WBCs	Must be compatible with recipient's plasma
FFP	Should be compatible with the recipient's RBCs
Cryoprecipitate	All ABO groups compatible
Platelets	All ABO groups acceptable; components compatible with recipient's RBCs are preferred

FFP, fresh frozen plasma; RBC, red blood cell; WBC, white blood cell.

- **Group B** antigen specificity confers an RBC with galactose on the RBC. Type B person produces antibodies to type A blood. Can receive type B or type O blood.
- **Group O** RBCs do not have A or B antigens; they may be transfused to all other ABO groups. Group O is the **universal donor**. Group O, however, has anti-A and anti-B antibodies because people with group O can receive only group O blood.
- **Group AB** is the **universal recipient** because people with group AB can receive any blood; they are lacking anti-A and anti-B antibodies.
- Plasma is given in the following way:
  - AB plasma may be transfused into any recipient.
  - Group O plasma can be given only to group O.
  - Group A or group B plasma is usually infused into ABO-identical recipients, or group O.

Platelets

■ Random Platelets: 50 mL

- Components in platelets:

1. More than 5.5×10^{10} platelets
2. RBCs
3. WBCs
4. Plasma
5. Cytokines

- Stored for 5 days, progressive loss in viability
- Stored at room temperature, risk of infection
- One unit of platelets expected to raise platelet count by 10,000/μL
- Usual dose: 4–6 units

■ Single-Donor Pheresis Platelets: 300 mL

- 3×10^{11} platelets, with same components as random platelets
- One unit expected to raise platelet count 30,000 to 50,000/μL
- Less exposure risk when coming from one donor
- Preferable to not give Rh-positive platelets to Rh-negative woman of childbearing age

■ Single-Donor Irradiated Filtered Platelets

- Safest platelets to give if patient will require repeated platelet transfusions
- Irradiated: to remove donor T cells and prevent graft-versus-host disease
- Leukocyte reduced: to remove leukocytes and leukocyte-produced cytokines

Fresh Frozen Plasma

- All coagulation factors, different half-lives
- Less than 12-hour half-life: factors V, VII, and VIII, protein C
- 12- to 24-hour half-life: factor IX and protein S
- 24- to 48-hour half-life: factor X
- More than 48-hour half-life: fibrinogen, factors XI, XII, and XIII, antithrombin
- 200 mL in the average size bag, on average 1 to 2 U/mL of clotting factors and 1 to 2 mg/mL of fibrinogen
- Should be ABO compatible

Cryoprecipitate

- Prepared by slow thawing fresh frozen plasma at 4° to 6°C
- Rich in factors: VIII, XIII, fibrinogen, von Willebrand factor
- Does not contain other coagulation factors

TRANSFUSION REACTIONS

Febrile Nonhemolytic Transfusion Reactions

- The most common reaction.
- Due to antibodies against the donor WBCs and HLA antigens.
- Symptoms: fever, chills, and rigors immediately or a few hours after transfusion.
- Treatment: slow transfusion in mild reaction; acetaminophen (Tylenol), diphenhydramine (Benadryl), or meperidine (Demerol) can be given.
- Prevent: leukocyte-reduced blood products.

Allergic Reactions

- Urticarial reactions.
- Due to plasma proteins.
- Symptoms: pruritic rash, edema, headache.
- Treatment: diphenhydramine, H_2-blocker, slow transfusion in mild cases, stop if severe.
- Prevent: premedicate for mild reactions, use washed blood products in future if severe.

Anaphylactic Reactions

- Severe reaction that occurs only after a few milliliters of blood products started.
- Reaction to plasma proteins.
- Commonly IgA-deficient individuals are susceptible. Also, patients who have PNH.
- Symptoms: coughing, nausea and emesis, dyspnea, bronchospasm, hypotension, shock, respiratory arrest, loss of consciousness.

■ Treatment
- Immediately stop the transfusion
- Maintain intravenous (IV) access
- Epinephrine 0.5–1.0 mg of 1:1000 IV stat
- Hydrocortisone 100 mg IV stat
- Use washed blood cell products or IgA-deficient plasma in the future

Acute Hemolytic Transfusion Reactions

- The recipient has preformed antibodies that bind and lyse donor RBCs.

- Usually the result of ABO incompatibility, which causes complement fixation on the RBC and lysis.
- Leads to intravascular hemolysis.
- Symptoms: fever, chills, tachycardia, tachypnea, back pain, chest pain, and general feeling of impending doom.
- Laboratory results: hemoglobinemia (red plasma) and hemoglobinuria (red urine), increased lactate dehydrogenase, increased total bilirubin, haptoglobin less than 10, positive direct Coombs test result.
- Acute renal failure and disseminated intravascular coagulation (DIC) can ensue.
- Treatment: Stop the transfusion.
- Maintain intravenous access.
- Start colloids and pressors if needed.
- Monitor urine output and for DIC.
- Order appropriate laboratory tests.
- Notify blood bank of error.
- Verify blood labels, paperwork, and patient identification.
- **Note: The most common reason for ABO incompatibility is clerical error.**

Delayed Hemolytic Transfusion Reactions

- Occurs in patients previously sensitized to RBC alloantigens.
- A negative alloantibody screen is due to low antibody levels.
- When the antigen-positive blood is transfused, the recipient immune cells produce antibodies that bind to donor RBCs.
- Usually an extravascular hemolysis, in distinction from an acute hemolytic transfusion reaction.
- The hemolytic reaction occurs 2 to 4 weeks after the transfusion; the Coombs antibody is detectable within 1 week.
- Previous pregnancies or previous transfusions are common.
- Laboratory results: increase in total bilirubin, LDH, positive Coombs test result.
- Treat: Check direct Coombs test and repeat compatibility tests.
- Transfuse with freshly cross-matched products.

Transfusion-Associated Graft-versus-Host Disease

- Donor T lymphocytes recognize host HLA antigens as foreign and mount an immune response.
- Symptoms: rash, elevated liver function test results and severe pancytopenia.

- Mortality is more than 80%.
- Seen in immunocompromised patients, patients taking immuno-suppressive medications, or immunocompetent patients who share HLA antigens with the donor.
- Resistant to most treatments.
- Prevention: Use irradiated blood products whenever possible.

Post-Transfusion Purpura

- One week after transfusion of any blood product.
- Rare, but bleeding can be life threatening.
- More common in multiparous women.
- Antibody to the platelet antigen HPA-1a that is lacking on the patient's platelets.
- Patient usually sensitized from prior exposure to blood products or pregnancy.
- Treatment: Only give HPA-1a–negative platelets; intravenous immunoglobulin and steroids.

Malignant Hematology

Acute Leukemia

Acute Myeloid Leukemia

- Malignancy of hematopoietic precursor cells of nonlymphoid lineage

Epidemiology

- Incidence: 3.5 cases per 100,000 population/yr.
- Leading cause of cancer deaths in adults younger than 35 years.
- The incidence of acute myeloid leukemia (AML) in adults is much higher than that of acute lymphocytic leukemia (ALL).
- AML accounts for 80% of all acute leukemia in adults.
- AML occurs with increased frequency as age advances.

Etiology

- Unclear
- Association with heavy radiation exposure; post-Chernobyl survivors
- Chronic benzene exposure
- Alkylating chemotherapy agents
- Genetic disorders: Down syndrome, Fanconi anemia, neurofibromatosis
- Pre-existing myeloproliferative disorders

Classification (Table 14-1)

Prognosis

- Younger age is favorable.
- Favorable risk cytogenetics: t(8;21), inv(16), t(15;17).
- Intermediate risk cytogenetics: normal diploidy.
- Poor risk cytogenetics: del(11q23) rearrangements; occurs after exposure to topoisomerase-2 inhibitors such as etoposide.
- Abnormality of chromosome 5 or 7: Often occurs in patients receiving alkylating agents previously or arising out of pre-existing myelodysplasia.
- Trisomy 8: Most common unfavorable genetic abnormality.

TABLE 14-1 Acute Myelogenous Leukemia		
Subtype	Morphologic (FAB)	Cytogenetics
M0	Minimally differentiated	t(8;21)
M1	Without maturation	t(8;21)
M2	With maturation	t(8;21)
M3	Promyelocytic leukemia	t(15;17)
M4	Myelomonocytic	inv(16)
M5	Monocytic	del(11q)
M6	Erythroleukemic	
M7	Megakaryocytic	

Acute myelogenous leukemia arising in setting of myelodysplasia or secondary to chemotherapy and/or radiation.
FAB, French-American British classification.
Italics indicate a distinct type of leukemia with excellent prognosis and special treatment.

- Untreated, AML is a fatal disease with a median survival of 3 months.
- Treated, 60% of newly diagnosed leukemics achieve complete remission.
- Median duration of first remission is 15 months and is dependent on subtype, cytogenetics, and age of patient.

■ Diagnosis

History and Physical Examination

- Peripheral smear shows characteristic blasts, usually with granules. Auer rods (rod-shaped cytoplasm inclusions) are indicative of AML and are a distinguishing feature from ALL.
- Failure of normal hematopoiesis causes most of the symptoms.
- Anemia: fatigue, malaise for several months, pallor, shortness of breath, tachycardia.
- Thrombocytopenia: easy bruising, bleeding, gum bleeding with tooth brushing, nosebleeds, and purpura on skin and in oral mucosa and palate.
- Neutropenia: fever, infection, particularly upper and lower respiratory tract infections.
- General: malaise, sweats, weight loss, and anorexia.
- Leukemia cutis (leukemic skin infiltration), Sweet syndrome (erythematous plaques infiltrated by neutrophils), pyoderma gangrenosum (ulcerative disease of the skin), and gum infiltration (more common in monocytic variants).
- Central nervous system disease: monocytic variants of AML. Headache, cranial nerve palsies (cranial nerves V and VII),

> ### ■ BOX 14-1 Diagnostic Workup
>
> - Labs: complete blood cell count, disseminated intravascular coagulation panel (international normalized ratio, activated partial thromboplastin time, fibrinogen, D-dimer)
> - Chemistry panel, uric acid, lactate dehydrogenase, liver panel
> - Blood cultures and urine cultures for fever
> - Chest radiograph
> - Multiple-gated acquisition scan or echocardiogram to evaluate ejection fraction
> - Bone marrow biopsy and aspirate with cytogenetics
> - Computed tomographic scan of head if neurologic symptoms
> - Lumbar puncture discouraged because it can cause seeding of spinal fluid

and ocular symptoms can be seen. Intracerebral masses are rare.
- Diagnostic workup is shown in Box 14-1.

■ Treatment

Hematologic Emergencies Associated with Leukemia

DISSEMINATED INTRAVASCULAR COAGULATION

- Common in acute promyelocytic leukemia (APL). Disseminated intravascular coagulation (DIC) can manifest in any leukemia and should be screened for in every patient.
- Pathophysiology: Release of tissue factor–like procoagulants from the azurophilic granules within the leukemia cells.
- Diligent and aggressive blood product support is the treatment for DIC in leukemia. Particular to APL is the institution of all-trans retinoic acid (ATRA). ATRA improves DIC in approximately 48 hours.
- Aminocaproic acid is an antifibrinolytic agent for treatment of isolated primary fibrinolysis. Heparin or low-molecular-weight heparins can be used to treat DIC.
- Tests to order and intervention for DIC are given in Table 14-2.

HYPERLEUKOCYTOSIS

- Defined as blood blast count of more than 100,000. The exact number of blasts to trigger aggressive treatment is controversial. If the patient is symptomatic, most recommend starting treatment regardless of absolute blast count.
- Pathophysiology: Blast cells are larger and more "sticky" in the circulation, leading to stasis and mimicking thrombosis.
- Leukostasis can occur anywhere, most common in the pulmonary, CNS, and genitourinary (GU) tract.

■ **TABLE 14-2 Disseminated Intravascular Coagulation Tests and Interventions**

Tests	Intervention
INR prolonged	FFP until normal
aPTT prolonged	FFP until normal
Fibrinogen low	Cryoprecipitate
Platelets low	Single-donor irradiated filtered platelets to keep count at greater than 50,000 μl

Other options include aminocaproic acid, low-dose heparin, and low-molecular-weight heparin. aPTT, activated partial thromboplastin time; FFP, fresh frozen plasma; INR, international normalized ratio.

■ **BOX 14-2 Treatment of Leukocytosis:**

- Leukophoresis if symptomatic or more than 100,000.
- Hydroxyurea at high doses.
- Allopurinol.
- Alkalinize the urine with bicarbonate added to the intravenously administered fluids.
- Minimize red blood cell transfusion to prevent further increases in viscosity.
- Start chemotherapy in prompt time frame.

- Pulmonary leukostasis: dyspnea, tachypnea, rales, respiratory failure.
- CNS leukostasis: headache, blurred vision, stroke symptoms with focal weakness.
- GU leukostasis: priapism, enlarged kidneys, hyperuricemia, renal failure.
- Pseudo-hyperkalemia, hypoglycemia, hypoxemia.
- Treatment is outlined in Box 14-2.

Chemotherapy
- Chemotherapy is divided into induction treatment and postinduction treatment:
  - Induction treatment: initial treatment to produce a remission. The blood counts return to within the normal reference range, and a bone marrow biopsy and aspirate is performed to document less than 5% blasts.
  - Postinduction treatment: Without more treatment, the relapse rate is 100%. The purpose of postinduction therapy is to eliminate the residual leukemia not detectable by standard means.

Other words used to describe this phase of treatment are consolidation or intensification.

- Maintenance: treatment that is ongoing, for 1 to 2 years after treatment.
- The most commonly used induction regimen for AML is the "7 and 3 regimen," a combination of 7 days of cytosine arabinoside and 3 days of an anthracycline.
- Postinduction therapy usually consists of high-dose cytosine arabinoside for two to three cycles.
- Bone marrow transplants are considered in patients with poor prognostic factors, such as poor cytogenetic AML. There are many types of transplant, including from a sibling (allogeneic), from a matched unrelated donor (MUD), or from the patient themselves (autologous). Also, there are many sources of stem cells, for example, peripheral blood is the most common, bone marrow in cases in which peripheral blood collection is scant, and in research settings, where umbilical cord blood is attempted.

Acute Promyelocytic Leukemia

■ Epidemiology

- Constitutes approximately 1% of cases on AML
- Can occur at any age, more common in younger patients
- Occurs with greater frequency among Latinos

■ Etiology

- Distinct subtype of AML characterized by a balanced translocation between chromosomes 15 and 17.
- On chromosome 17 is the retinoic acid receptor gene (RAR-α); 17q21.
- On chromosome 15 is the promyelocytic leukemia (PML) gene; 15q24.
- The translocation forms an abnormal hybrid fusion gene, PML/RAR-α, which encodes a protein that blocks myeloid differentiation. This leads to an accumulation of abnormal promyelocytes (promyelocyte arrest) in the bone marrow.

■ Classification

- Identified by the French-American-British classification as AML-M3.
- Microgranular variant can be confused with monocytic leukemia (M5).

- Identification is by the t(15;17) in the peripheral blood or bone marrow.

■ Prognosis

- Excellent prognosis with approximately 80% being cured with treatment.
- Highest risk of relapse is seen in patients with higher white blood cell (WBC) counts; greater than 10×10^9/L.
- Patients 30 years or younger have a better chance of cure.

■ Diagnosis

- The same diagnostic workup holds for APL.
- The t(15;17) is the identifying abnormality and is present virtually 100% of the time.
- Peripheral smear shows characteristic promyelocytes and faggot (cord of wood) cells (collection of Auer rods in a bundle).

History and Physical Examination

- Much greater propensity to bleed due to DIC and increased fibrinolysis.
- Bleeding can be fatal. Patients can present with fatal intracranial bleeds, hemoptysis, hematuria, vaginal bleeding, or skin and mucous membrane bleeding.
- DIC panel should be checked and treated with prompt aggressive replacement of blood products.

■ Treatment

- ATRA is a medication used in APL with excellent responses.
- ATRA binds to PML/RAR-α, downregulating the abnormal hybrid gene.
- Downregulation of the gene causes terminal differentiation of APL blasts.
- Blasts then differentiate to neutrophils and the DIC risk subsides in approximately 48 hours.
- Thus, ATRA causes a maturing of the leukemic cells and stops the coagulopathy.
- Approximately 80% of patients respond to this treatment and are cured of their leukemia, whereas the other 20% of patients who die with APL do so from DIC complications or relapsing resistant disease.
- ATRA induction is followed by several cycles of anthracycline-based consolidation chemotherapy.

- Salvage therapy involves arsenic trioxide, high doses of cytotoxic chemotherapy followed by autologous (from oneself), allogeneic (from a sibling), or MUD transplantation.

Acute Lymphocytic Leukemia

- Malignancy of hematopoietic precursor cells of lymphoid lineage

■ Epidemiology

- ALL is the most common malignancy in children ages 2 to 10 years.
- Comprises only 20% of adult leukemia cases.
- 1 in 70,000 annually, AML is seven times more common than ALL.

■ Etiology

- Unclear
- Association with heavy radiation exposure; post-Chernobyl survivors
- Chronic benzene exposure
- Genetic disorders: Down syndrome, Fanconi anemia, neurofibromatosis

■ Classification (Table 14-3)

■ TABLE 14-3 Acute Lymphocytic Leukemia Classification

Morphological

L1	Small blasts with single nucleolus
L2	Larger blasts
L3	Largest blasts with vacuoles, called Burkitt type

Immunophenotyping
Lymphocyte markers differentiate early pre-B-cell ALL, pre-B-cell ALL, null-cell ALL. T-cell phenotype is rare, and fewer than 10% are T cell.

Cytogenetic Finding	Genetic Alteration	Prognosis
t(9:22)	*BCR/ABL*	*Unfavorable*
t(4:11)	AF4/MLL	Unfavorable
t(1:19)	PBX/E2A	Unfavorable
t(12:21)	TEL/AML1	Favorable
Hyperdiploidy		Favorable

Italics indicates Philadelphia-positive t(9;22) ALL, which connotes a very poor prognosis.
ALL, acute lymphocytic leukemia.

■ **Prognosis**

ALL Favorable Prognostic Features
- Age younger than 60 years
- WBC count less than 30,000
- T-cell phenotype
- Hyperdiploidy
- Mediastinal mass
- Absence of t(9;22), t(4;11), or t(18;14)

■ **Diagnosis**
- Same diagnostic workup as AML (see Box 14-1).
- Peripheral smear indicates characteristic lymphoblasts. Auer rods and granules are not seen in ALL.
- Failure of normal hematopoiesis causes most of the symptoms.
- Anemia: fatigue, malaise for several months, pallor, shortness of breath, tachycardia.
- Thrombocytopenia: easy bruising, bleeding, gum bleeding with tooth brushing, nosebleeds, and purpura on skin and in oral mucosa and palate.
- Neutropenia: fever, infection, particularly upper and lower respiratory tract infections.
- General: malaise, sweats, weight loss, and anorexia.
- Widespread lymphadenopathy: more common in ALL, mild to moderate splenomegaly, hepatomegaly.
- Leukemic skin infiltration, called leukemia cutis, Sweet syndrome, pyoderma gangrenosum, gum infiltration (more common in monocytic variants of AML).
- CNS disease: Meningeal disease in 15% of adults with ALL, headache or cranial nerve palsies (cranial nerves V and V11), ocular symptoms, and intracerebral masses are rare.

■ **Treatment**
- ALL regimens are complicated and involve many cytotoxic chemotherapy combinations.
- The treatment is divided into several phases: induction, early intensification, CNS prophylaxis, late intensification, and maintenance.
- Incidence of CNS relapse is much higher in ALL than in AML necessitating CNS prophylaxis.
- Induction chemotherapy medications include cyclophosphamide, anthracyclines, vincristine, and steroids.
- Early intensification therapy includes cyclophosphamide, 6-mercaptopurine, cytarabine, vincristine, and asparaginase.
- CNS prophylaxis: intrathecal methotrexate or other chemotherapeutics.

- Late intensification therapy includes anthracyclines, vincristine, steroids, cyclophosphamide, 6-thioguanine, and cytarabine.
- Prolonged maintenance therapy includes vincristine, prednisone, 6-mercatopurine, and methotrexate.
- Bone marrow transplants are considered in patients will poor prognostic factors, such as Philadelphia positive t(9;22) ALL and relapsed disease. As stated earlier, there are many types of transplants: from a sibling (allogeneic), from an MUD, or from the patient him or herself (autologous).

Chronic Leukemias

Chronic Lymphocytic Leukemia

■ Epidemiology

- Most common adult leukemia in Western Hemisphere
- Median age at diagnosis is 60 years
- Slight male predominance (2:1)
- Not associated with radiation exposure
- Familial cases reported more frequently

■ Pathophysiology

- **Peripheral blood lymphocytosis** with variable degrees of lymph node, spleen, liver, and bone marrow involvement.
- More than 95% are of B-cell origin.
- Two subtypes are now recognized: nonmutated and mutated chronic lymphocytic leukemia (CLL).
  - **Nonmutated CLL:** pregerminal naive B cell that has *not* undergone somatic mutation of the immunoglobulin variable (V) region of the heavy-chain genes. Somatic mutation generally occurs after B cells are exposed to antigen in the germinal center of the lymph nodes. Thus, nonmutated CLL is a naive B cell and connotes a *worse prognosis*.
  - **Mutated CLL:** memory B cell that has undergone somatic mutation of the immunoglobulin variable (V) heavy-chain genes. V gene hypermutation is consistent with a post–germinal center memory B cell. Thus, mutated CLL is a B cell that has already encountered antigen and confers a much better prognosis for the patient.

■ Clinical Manifestations

- Usually picked up early due to an elevated white blood cell (WBC) count with predominant lymphocytosis.
- B symptoms: fever, night sweats, weight loss, fatigue.
- Frequent infections, organomegaly (splenomegaly, hepatomegaly), lymphadenopathy, autoimmune complications, and symptoms related to cytopenias.

- Lymphadenopathy: usually cervical, axillary, or inguinal areas.
- Symptoms of leukostasis are very uncommon, and patients with very high WBC counts can be entirely asymptomatic.

■ Complications

- Increased risk of autoimmune phenomenon: idiopathic thrombocytopenia purpura (ITP), autoimmune hemolytic anemia, pure red cell aplasia, neutropenia
- Increased risk of autoimmune disorders: rheumatoid arthritis, thyroid disorders, and systemic lupus erythematosus
- Increased risk of secondary malignancies
- Infectious complications
- Hypogammaglobulinemia; check quantitative immunoglobulins

■ Diagnosis

- Complete blood count and review of peripheral smear: Lymphocytosis is defined as more than 5×10^9/L. Evaluate for anemia (order direct Coombs test), thrombocytopenia, and neutropenia. Smear shows mature predominance of lymphocytes with some smudge cells (damaged fragile CLL cells).
- Flow cytometry: Exclusively kappa or lambda light chain proves clonality. Immunophenotype: commonly CD5+, CD19+, CD20+ (dim), CD23+, dim surface immunoglobulin (Table 15-1).

■ Staging

- Two proposed classic staging systems (Tables 15-2 and 15-3)
- Bone marrow biopsy and aspirate: indicated before starting therapy; not necessary to make diagnosis; nodular infiltration preferable to diffuse infiltration

■ TABLE 15-1 Flow Cytometry Patterns

		CD20	CD5	CD10	CD23	CD43	Surface Ig	Cyclin D$_1$
CLL	[TB]+		++	––	++	++	+	+/–
LPL	[TB]++		–	––	––	+/–	++	–
MCL	[TB]++		++	––	––	++	++	++
MZL	[TB]++		––	––	––	+/–	++	––
FCL	[TB]++		––	60%+	––	––	++	––
HCL	[TB]++		––	––	––	+/–	++	––

CLL, chronic lymphocytic leukemia; FCL, follicular lymphoma (leukemic phase); HCL, hairy cell leukemia; Ig, immunoglobulin; LPL, lymphoplasmacytic lymphoma; MCL, mantle cell lymphoma; MZL, marginal zone Lymphoma.

■ TABLE 15-2 Rai Staging

Stage	Median Survival (yr)
0 Lymphocytosis alone	14.5
1 Lymphocytosis, lymphadenopathy	7.5
2 Lymphocytosis, hepatosplenomegaly	7.5
3 Lymphocytosis, anemia (hemoglobin < 11 g/dL)	2.5
4 Lymphocytosis, thrombocytopenia <100,000/µL)	2.5

■ TABLE 15-3 Binet Staging

Stage	Median Survival (yr)
A Lymphocytosis, fewer than three areas of lymphadenopathy	14.0
B Lymphocytosis, three or more areas of lymphadenopathy	5.0
C Anemia, thrombocytopenia	2.5

- Cytogenetics: conventional cytogenetics testing difficult in CLL because the cells are not rapidly dividing
- Fluorescence *in situ* hybridization (FISH):
  - Favorable FISH: 13q–, normal karyotype
  - Unfavorable FISH: 17p–, 11q–, trisomy 12

■ Prognostic Markers

- CD38-positive surface antigen (detected by flow cytometry) is an unfavorable marker.
- Elevated β_2-microglobulin is an unfavorable marker.
- Nonmutated variable heavy-chain genes are unfavorable and technically very difficult to test.
- Lymphocyte doubling time (LDT) less than 12 months is unfavorable.
- Zeta-associated Protein-70 (ZAP-70), a tyrosine kinase involved in T-cell signaling, appears to be correlated with mutated versus nonmutated status. A low expression of ZAP-70 on flow cytometry confers a mutated status and thus longer survival.

■ Treatment

National Cancer Institute Criteria for Treatment
- Worsening anemia (<10.5 g/dL) or thrombocytopenia (<100 × 10^9/L) due to marrow failure.
- More than 50% increase in absolute lymphocyte count in less than 2 months or anticipated LDT of less than 6 months.
- Progressive or massive splenomegaly or lymphadenopathy.

- "B" symptoms include weight loss, fever, night sweats, extreme fatigue.
- Autoimmune anemia or ITP is poorly responsive to steroids.
- Patients with unfavorable FISH results, CD38+, elevated β_2-microglobulin, and nonmutated heavy-chain gene and who are ZAP-70 positive probably mandate earlier treatment as well.
- A new paradigm in hematology will be relying on FISH, flow cytometry results, and other prognostic molecular markers over the classic clinical intuition.

Richter Transformation
- Rapid enlargement in lymph nodes, acutely worsening B symptoms
- Consider that patient may have transformed to an aggressive histology and now mandates new excisional nodal biopsy

Treatment Options
- Keep in mind that CLL is not curable.
- CLL tends to be chronic and minimally symptomatic for years.
- Patients should be treated when symptoms become apparent or worsen.
- Fludarabine alone has a 70% response rate; test for direct Coombs because fludarabine may aggravate autoimmune hemolytic anemia
- Chlorambucil has a 35% response rate, overall the same as fludarabine. Can convert to fludarabine when needed; it is not advised to administer chlorambucil after fludarabine treatment because the duration of response is minimal. This is a good treatment for elderly patients or poor performance status patients.
- Fludarabine combinations: with Cytoxan, with rituxan, or with Cytoxan and rituxan—known as FCR regimen. These immunocompromising treatments are associated with infections. Patients should be placed on prophylaxis for *Pneumocystis carinii* pneumonia with trimethoprim-sulfamethoxazole (Bactrim) and for herpes with acyclovir and for fungal infections with fluconazole. Cytomegalovirus (CMV) should be in the differential for fever in patients treated with fludarabine.
- Alemtuzumab, a monoclonal antibody for refractory CLL, targets the CD52 on B and T cells and is highly immunosuppressive. Consider CMV in patients presenting with fever treated with alemtuzumab.
- Stem cell transplant: Consider transplant for younger patients with aggressive or recurrent disease.
- Immunize patients for pneumococcus and influenza infection. Patients should be offered intravenous immunoglobulin (IVIg) for recurrent infections and/or hypogammaglobulinemia.

Chronic Myeloid Leukemia

■ Epidemiology

- Chronic myeloid leukemia (CML) represents 15% of all leukemias; incidence is 1.6 per 100,000 population.
- Median age at diagnosis (depending on reports) is about 55 years.
- Affects men slightly more than women, 1.4:1.0.

■ Risk Factors

- There is no known genetic predisposition or chemical exposure related to CML.

■ Pathogenesis

- 90% of patients have the "Philadelphia chromosome," an acquired translocation between chromosomes 9 and 22 t(9;22), which results in the Bcr/Abl fusion protein.
- The fusion protein results in constitutive expression of **tyrosine kinase,** leading to dysregulated cell growth, differentiation, and apoptosis.
- The Ph chromosome is not pathognomonic; it is also found in 25% to 50% of patients with ALL, 2% of patients with AML, and even some healthy individuals!

■ Clinical Manifestations

History

- Clinical course involves three phases.

CHRONIC (STABLE) PHASE

- 90% of patients present in this phase, often with nonspecific symptoms such as fatigue, weight loss, early satiety, or bone pain.
- 50% of patients are asymptomatic (i.e., the disease is detected incidentally).
- 50% of patients have splenomegaly, WBC count more than 100, anemia, or a few blasts in the periphery; 15% present with increased basophils in the periphery.
- This phase generally lasts 3 to 8 years.
- Only 5% to 10% of patients transform to the blastic phase in the first 2 years.
- 25% of patients will skip the accelerated phase and transform to blastic.
- Without treatment, 100% ultimately progress to the blastic phase.

ACCELERATED PHASE

The accelerated phase usually lasts 3 to 18 months. There are three sets of criteria for diagnosing this phase; we'll use the MD Anderson model:

- Platelets less than 100,000
- Peripheral blasts more than 15%
- Blasts + promyelocytes 30% or more
- Basophils more than 20%
- Karyotypic evolution: 50% to 80% of patients will acquire additional chromosomal changes, the most common being trisomy 8.

BLASTIC PHASE

- Patients often present with fever, weight loss, anemia, and bleeding.
- Diagnosis is confirmed by the presence of 20% or more blasts in the marrow or peripheral blood or by extramedullary (outside the bone marrow) blastic infiltrates.
- One third of patients will express the lymphoid markers CD19, CD20, or CD10 on their blasts; they have better prognoses and respond to therapies used for ALL.
- Two thirds of patients' blasts will be myeloid; they have poorer prognoses and respond to the therapies used for AML.

■ Diagnostic Evaluation

- Start with a complete blood cell count with differential.
- For patients with a moderately elevated WBC count of uncertain etiology, a low leukocyte alkaline phosphatase blood level suggests that it is not a response to infection.
- Next, perform bone marrow biopsy and aspiration looking for blasts.
- Search for the Ph chromosome.
- **Cytogenetic analysis** is the gold standard for detecting the Ph chromosome, but it is time consuming and fails in 10% of patients. Genomic studies, with polymerase chain reaction (PCR) and **Southern blot,** can detect exact breakpoints of fusion genes.
- Reverse transcriptase PCR and **Northern blot** can detect Bcr-Abl transcripts at the RNA level but may miss those who are not actively transcribing the gene.
- **Western blot** or immunoprecipitation demonstrate the transcription protein using monoclonal antibodies.
- **FISH** allows analysis of nondividing interphase and metaphase cells and is easily quantifiable.

■ Treatment and Prognosis

- There are three concepts to the treatment of CML:
  - **Hematologic control:** Maintain cell counts in normal range without changing the natural progression of the disease or affecting Ph positivity; for example, hydroxyurea, a DNA synthesis inhibitor, or the older drug busulfan.
  - **Cytogenetic remission:** loss (or at least significant reduction) of Ph with improved survival; for example, interferon-α (or PEG-IFN) plus/minus cytarabine and now, even better, STI 571 (Gleevec), a tyrosine kinase inhibitor that is taken by mouth and is highly effective short term (studies on durability of response are in progress).
  - **Cure:** The only proven "cure" is stem cell transplant and the best statistics are achieved with a matched sibling donor (50% 10-year survival), in patients younger than 30 years who are CMV negative and who are early in the chronic phase (aim for <2 years).
- Estimated median survival for patients in the chronic phase on IFN is 7 to 9 years.
- For patients in the accelerated phase with stem cell transplant, the 5-year survival is 20% to 40%.
- For patients in the blastic phase with stem cell transplant, the 5-year survival is 0% to 25%.

16 Lymphomas

The two main groups of lymphomas are non-Hodgkin lymphoma (NHL) and Hodgkin disease (HD), which are discussed separately for ease of understanding.

Non-Hodgkin Lymphoma

■ Epidemiology

- In the year 2004, 53,370 Americans will be diagnosed with NHL, 28,850 men and 25,520 women.
- Incidence rates for NHL have nearly doubled since the 1970s.
- NHL incidence is highest in the United States and developed countries, with the exception of western Africa.
- Lymphoma is increased substantially in the acquired immunodeficiency syndrome (AIDS) population.

■ Pathogenesis

- An infectious etiology of lymphoid malignancies has been borne out for many lymphomas (Table 16-1).

■ Histopathology and Classification

Non-Hodgkin's Lymphoma World Health Organization (WHO)/REAL Classification

LOW-GRADE LYMPHOMAS
- B-cell lymphomas:
  1. Small lymphocytic lymphoma/B-cell chronic lymphocytic leukemia (CLL)
  2. Lymphoplasmacytic lymphoma (Waldenström lymphoma)
  3. Plasma cell lymphoma/plasmacytoma
  4. Hairy cell leukemia
  5. Follicular lymphoma (grades I and II)
  6. Marginal zone B-cell lymphoma
  7. Mantle cell lymphoma
- T-cell lymphomas:
  1. T-cell large granular lymphocytic lymphoma
  2. Mycosis fungoides
  3. T-cell prolymphocytic leukemia

■ **TABLE 16-1 Lymphoma Subtypes Linked to Infectious Agents**

Lymphoma	Agent
Mucosal-associated lymphoid tissue	*Helicobacter pylori*
Burkitt lymphoma	EBV
Hodgkin disease	EBV
Post-transplant lymphoproliferative disease	EBV
AIDS-related NHL	HIV
Adult T-cell leukemia/lymphoma	HTLV-1
Primary effusion lymphoma	HHV-8
Lymphoplasmacytic lymphoma	Hepatitis C
Mediterranean lymphoma	Intestinal pathogen

AIDS, acquired immunodeficiency syndrome; EBV, Epstein-Barr virus; HHV-8, human herpesvirus-8; HIV, human immunodeficiency virus; HTLV-1, human T-cell leukemia virus; NHL, non-Hodgkin lymphoma.

- **Natural-killer (NK) cell lymphomas/leukemias:**
  1. NK cell large granular lymphocyte leukemia

INTERMEDIATE GRADE LYMPHOMAS
- **B-cell lymphomas:**
  1. Follicular (grade III) lymphoma
  2. Diffuse large B-cell lymphoma
- **T-cell lymphomas:**
  1. Peripheral T-cell lymphoma
  2. Anaplastic large cell lymphoma

HIGH-GRADE LYMPHOMAS
- **B-cell lymphomas:**
  1. Burkitt lymphoma
  2. Precursor B lymphoblastic leukemia/lymphoma
- **T-cell lymphomas:**
  1. Adult T-cell lymphoma/leukemia
  2. Precursor T lymphoblastic leukemia/lymphoma

■ **Clinical Manifestations**

Low-Grade Lymphomas
- Slow growing, but paradoxically incurable with current therapy.
- Widely disseminated at diagnosis but follows indolent course.
- 40% of cases of lymphoma are low grade.
- Common in middle age to elderly; median age is 55 years.
- 66% of patients present with stage III or IV disease.

- Median survival is 10 years.
- 30% of low-grade lymphomas may transform to a more aggressive histology.

Intermediate Grade Lymphomas

- Diffuse large B-cell lymphomas represent approximately 50% of NHL cases; the most common histology.
- Presents with stage I or II disease in more than half of patients.
- Rapidly growing lymphoma that can be curable with current therapy.
- Short history of localized rapidly enlarging lymphadenopathy and constitutional symptoms.
- Median survival varies from 3 to 4 years depending on subtype.

High-Grade Lymphoma

- Approximately 10% of NHL cases.
- Younger patients with aggressive fast-growing lymphomas needing prompt treatment.
- High-grade lymphomas, especially Burkitt lymphoma, have the fastest doubling times of any tumors.
- B- and T-cell lymphoblastic lymphomas share features of acute lymphocytic leukemia (ALL).
- Median survival is less than 2 years.
- Patients likely to present with tumor lysis, rapidly enlarging lymph nodes, constitutional symptoms, and need hospitalization.

▪ Staging

1. Stage I: disease involving a single lymph node region or a single extralymphatic organ or site (stage IE)
2. Stage II: disease involving two or more involved lymph node regions on the same side of the diaphragm or with localized involvement of an extralymphatic organ or site (stage IIE)
3. Stage III: disease involving lymph nodes on both sides of the diaphragm or with localized involvement of an extralymphatic organ or site (stage IIIE), spleen (stage IIIS), or both (stage IIIES)
4. Stage IV: presence of diffuse or disseminated involvement of one or more extralymphatic organ (liver, bone marrow, lung), with or without associated lymphadenopathy

▪ Physical Examination

- Examination of all lymph node sites
- Waldeyer ring; tonsils, base of tongue, nasopharynx
- Standard lymph node sites: cervical, supraclavicular, axillary, inguinal, femoral

- Liver and spleen
- Less commonly involved sites: occipital, preauricular, epitrochlear
- Careful skin examination in patients presenting with T-cell lymphoma

■ Laboratory Features

- Rarely cytopenias, only if extensive bone marrow involvement.
- Normochromic, normocytic anemia.
- Hyperuricemia may develop and cause symptoms of gout or nephrolithiasis.
- Lactate dehydrogenase (LDH) may be elevated; indicator of bulky disease.
- Alkaline phosphatase may be increased with bone or liver involvement.
- Peripheral blood may rarely show lymphoma cells in high-grade disease.

■ Workup

1. History and physical (H&P)
2. Lymph node biopsy: better to perform excisional biopsy (remove entire lymph node) for accurate assessment of architecture by pathologist
3. Peripheral smear review
4. Complete blood cell (CBC) count, complete chemistry panel, liver function tests, LDH, and uric acid
5. Human immunodeficiency virus (HIV) testing, hepatitis B and C testing, and appropriate infectious testing depending on type of lymphoma; for example, *Helicobacter pylori* in mucosal-associated lymphoid tissue (MALT) lymphoma
6. Bone marrow biopsy and aspirate with cytogenetics and flow cytometry
7. Computed tomographic (CT) scan of chest, abdomen, and pelvis
8. Positron emission tomographic (PET) scan of body
9. Lumbar puncture in some cases

■ Prognostic Factors

- Histological grade: variable and highly dependent on subtype.
- Age younger than 60 years: favorable prognosis.
- Performance status: Advanced status indicates a poor prognosis.
- Increased LDH: unfavorable prognosis.
- Bulky disease (>10 cm): unfavorable prognosis.
- Extranodal disease: unfavorable prognosis.
- Increased LDH: unfavorable prognosis.

■ TABLE 16-2 International Prognostic Index		
	Five-Year Survival	
Risk	Age <60 yr	Age >60 yr
Low risk: score of zero to one	83%	56%
Low intermediate risk: score of two	69%	44%
High intermediate risk: score of three	46%	37%
High risk: score of four or five	32%	21%

International Prognostic Index (Table 16-2)
- Originally developed in patients with intermediate and high-grade NHL.
- One point is given for each of the following:
  - Age older than 60 years
  - LDH greater than normal
  - Poor performance status
  - Stage III or IV disease
  - Number of involved extranodal sites more than one

■ **Treatment**

Low-Grade Disease
- Watch and wait: no advantage to starting treatment on survival if patient is asymptomatic
- Chemotherapy: fludarabine, Cytoxan, rituxan, Cytoxan-vincristine-prednisone (CVP)
- Radiation: local control or in limited stage disease
- Relapse: many chemotherapy options, radiolabeled antibodies

Intermediate Grade
- Standard of care for many years was CHOP (Cytoxan-adriamyacin-vincristine-prednisone).
- Rituxan: monoclonal antibody directed against CD20 expressed on all B cells and B-cell lymphomas.
- Radiation: local control or early stage disease.
- Relapse: autologous stem cell transplant.

High Grade
- ALL regimen complicated chemotherapy necessitating hospitalization

Hodgkin Disease

■ **Epidemiology**
- HD will be diagnosed in 7880 patients: 3550 in women, 4330 in men.

- Incidence rates for HD have declined since the 1970s.
- A distinguishing feature of HD is the bimodal age distribution incidence peaks: one in young adults and one in older age.

■ Pathogenesis
- Epstein-Barr virus (EBV) has been linked to the development of HD.

■ Classifications
Four Subtypes
1. Nodular sclerosis (NS): onset at a young age (15 to 30 years), more often in men, involvement of mediastinal nodes common, limited disease frequently
2. Mixed cellularity (MC): intermediate prognosis, onset at an older age, common to have B symptoms, extensive disease
3. Lymphocyte depleted (LD): poor prognosis, presents in elderly, extensive disease
4. Lymphocyte predominant (LP): distinct clinical subtype, excellent prognosis, limited disease

■ Clinical Manifestations
- Painless lymph node enlargement above the diaphragm.
- Usually involves the cervical lymph nodes.
- Lymph nodes that wax and wane are not an uncommon finding.
- Abdominal involvement is unusual without splenic involvement.
- The spleen in involved approximately 30% of the time.
- Characterized by orderly spread from one lymph node region to contiguous nodal sites.
- Bone lesions appear osteoblastic on radiographs.
- Approximately 30% have "B" symptoms: drenching night sweats, fever, and weight loss.
- Pruritus is a common symptom.
- Pain induced by alcohol at sites of adenopathy.
- Can present with superior vena cava syndrome: cough, chest discomfort, local facial swelling.

■ Staging
- Stage I: disease involving a single lymph node region or a single extralymphatic organ or site (stage IE)
- Stage II: disease involving two or more involved lymph node regions on the same side of the diaphragm or with localized involvement of an extralymphatic organ or site (stage IIE)
- Stage III: disease involving lymph nodes on both sides of the diaphragm or with localized involvement of an extralymphatic organ or site (stage IIIE), spleen (stage IIIS), or both (stage IIIES)

- Stage IV: presence of diffuse or disseminated involvement of one or more extralymphatic organ (liver, bone marrow, lung), with or without associated lymphadenopathy
- A = absence of constitutional "B" symptoms
- B = drenching night sweats, fever, and weight loss.

■ Physical Examination

- Examination of all lymph node sites
- Waldeyer ring; tonsils, base of tongue, nasopharynx
- Standard lymph node sites: cervical, supraclavicular, axillary, inguinal, femoral
- Liver and spleen
- Less commonly involved sites: occipital, preauricular, epitrochlear

■ Laboratory Features

- Rarely cytopenias, only if extensive bone marrow involvement.
- Normochromic, normocytic anemia.
- Hyperuricemia may develop and cause symptoms of gout or nephrolithiasis.
- LDH may be elevated; indicator of bulky disease.
- Alkaline phosphatase may be increased with bone or liver involvement.
- Peripheral blood may rarely show lymphoma cells in high-grade disease.

■ Workup

1. H&P
2. Lymph node biopsy: better to perform excisional biopsy (remove entire lymph node) for accurate assessment of architecture by pathologist.
3. Peripheral smear review
4. CBC, complete chemistry panel, liver function tests, LDH, and uric acid
5. HIV testing, hepatitis B and C testing, and EBV serological testing
6. Bone marrow biopsy and aspirate with cytogenetics and flow cytometry
7. CT of chest, abdomen, pelvis
8. PET scan of body
9. Lumbar puncture in some cases

■ Prognostic Factors

- Favorable prognostic factors: age younger than 50 years, female, lumbar puncture, or NS histology, not more than three nodal areas involved.

■ Treatment

- 80% of all patients with HD are cured.
- The intent of treatment in every stage is always curative.
- Early stage: controversial, combination of chemotherapy and radiation or either modality alone.
- Chemotherapy is the standard of care for stage III and IV disease.
- ABVD is the standard chemo regimen; adriamycin, bleomycin, vinblastine, and dacarbazine.
- Other regimens for high-risk disease: BEACOPP and Stanford 5.
- Salvage therapy: Patients who relapse after treatment are commonly given high-dose chemotherapy and autologous stem cell transplant.
- Complications: increased risk of secondary tumors, sterility, increased risk of acute leukemia, bleomycin related pulmonary disease, and radiation-induced cardiopulmonary disease.

Myelodysplasia

- Acquired clonal disorders of bone marrow
- Dysplastic and ineffective blood cell production
- Hypercellular bone marrow
- Cells unable to mature normally, resulting in peripheral blood cytopenias
- Can progress to acute leukemia

■ Epidemiology

- Risk of myelodysplasia (MDS) increases with age, predominantly seen in older patients.
- Median age at diagnosis is 64 years.
- 4.1 per 100,000 is a rough annual incidence.
- Onset of MDS before age 50 years is unusual, except with treatment-induced MDS and among Asians.

■ Pathophysiology

- Ineffective hematopoiesis: formation of blood cells that are so defective (dysplastic) that they are destroyed in the bone marrow.
- Apoptosis (programmed cell death) of blood-forming cells is the major factor leading to pancytopenia in MDS.
- Apoptotic factors and mediators are increased in patients with MDS.
- Few cells do leave the bone marrow but are usually not functional.
- Platelets and leukocytes are many times dysfunctional, necessitating higher transfusion levels for platelets and careful attention to infection risk even with a normal neutrophil count.
- Hypercellularity in the bone marrow, possibly as an attempt to increase the rate of cells made to overcome intramedullary cell death.
- Chromosomal abnormalities are common in MDS.

■ Clinical Manifestations

- Relates to the predominant cytopenia.
- Anemia: fatigue, tiredness, tachycardia, malaise. Macrocytic anemia is commonly seen.

- Thrombocytopenia: bruising, bleeding. Functionally deficient platelets can cause symptoms even at a platelet count of 50,000/L.
- Neutropenia: infection. Patients are susceptible to infection even at normal neutrophil counts because of dysfunctional neutrophils.
- Constitutional symptoms: weight loss, night sweats, fever, malaise, and anorexia.
- Autoimmune phenomenon.
- Cutaneous manifestations: Sweet syndrome (fever and neutrophilic dermatosis), granulocytic sarcoma.

■ Diagnosis

Anemia
- Rule out other causes of anemia, especially vitamin B_{12} and folate deficiency anemia. Usually an inappropriately low reticulocyte count.

Peripheral Smear Findings
- Red blood cells (RBCs): macrocytes, nucleated RBCs, basophilic stippling, Howell-Jolly bodies
- White blood cells: pseudo–Pelger-Huët anomaly, Auer rods, hypogranulation, ring-shaped nuclei
- Platelets: giant platelets, hypogranular platelets

Bone Marrow Biopsy and Aspirate with Cytogenetics
- Hypercellularity with characteristic marrow abnormalities. Acquired cytogenetic abnormalities can be useful to prognosticate patients with MDS.

■ Classification (Table 17-1)

Therapy-Related MDS
- Exposure to alkylating agents, topoisomerase inhibitors, or radiation
- Alkylating agents: deletion in chromosome 5 and 7 common
- Topoisomerase inhibitors: 11q23 translocation
- Less favorable prognosis

■ Prognosis
- Table 17-2 outlines the international prognostic scoring system.

■ Treatment
- Mild cytopenias: observation
- Anemia: growth factors

■ TABLE 17-1 Myelodysplasia Classification

Disorder	Findings in Marrow
Refractory anemia	Erythroid dysplasia only
Refractory anemia with ringed sideroblasts	>15% ringed sideroblasts
Refractory cytopenia with multilineage dysplasia	Dysplasia in >10% of cells in two or more myeloid cell lines
Refractory cytopenia with multilineage dysplasia and ringed sideroblasts	>15% ringed sideroblasts
Refractory anemia with excess blasts-1	5% to 9% blasts
Refractory anemia with excess blasts-2	10% to 19% blasts
MDS unclassifiable	Unilineage dysplasia in granulocytes or megakaryocytes
MDS with del(5q)	Isolated del(5q)

MDS, myelodysplastic syndrome.

■ TABLE 17-2 International Prognostic Scoring System

Parameter	Criteria	Score
Blast count in bone marrow	<5%	0
	5% to 10%	0.5
	11% to 20%	1.5
	21% to 30%	2
Karyotype	Normal or 5q	0
	Other	0.5
	Three abnormalities or poor-prognosis ones	1.0
Cytopenias	None or one lineage	0
	Two or three lineages	0.5

Total score: 0, low risk, median survival 6 years; 0.5 to 1.0, intermediate risk 1, median survival 3.5 years; 1.5 to 2.0, intermediate risk 2, median survival 1.2 years; >2.5, high risk, median survival 0.4 years.

- Leukopenia: growth factors
- Thrombocytopenia: growth factors
- Chemotherapy
- Allogeneic or autologous transplant
- Investigational medications

18 Myeloproliferative Disorders

Chronic myeloproliferative disorders (CMDs) are classified into several subgroups:

1. Chronic myeloid leukemia (CML): discussed in Chapter 15
2. Polycythemia vera (PV)
3. Agnogenic myeloid metaplasia (AMM)
4. Essential thrombocythemia (ET)

■ Epidemiology

- Incidence is rare, approximately 2.5, 2.3, 1.3/100,000 for ET, PV, and AMM, respectively.
- Main incidence is 50 to 79 years of age.
- Slight male predominance in PV and AMM.
- Age-specific female predominance at 30 to 50 years of age in ET.
- Identified with increasing frequency as a result of routine complete blood cell (CBC) counts.

■ Pathophysiology

- Clonal stem cell disorder
- All hematopoietic cell lines are affected, with frequent predominance of one cell line. For example, platelets are commonly elevated in ET; hemoglobin is commonly elevated in PV.

Agnogenic Myeloid Metaplasia

- Distinct clinical form of the CMD.
- A clonal disorder affecting all hematopoietic cell lines, although it is also associated with extensive marrow fibrosis.
- Characterized by "extramedullary hematopoiesis," the forming of hematopoietic stem cells outside of the bone marrow.
- Because of the extensive fibrosis and marrow "gridlock," the stem cells migrate out of the marrow to fetal hematopoietic organs (spleen and liver and occasionally other locations). This results in hepatosplenomegaly.
- The "reactive" fibrosis in the marrow is not derived from the same clone.

■ Clinical Manifestations

Polycythemia Vera

HISTORY

- Explore secondary causes of elevated hemoglobin: tobacco use, alcohol use, obesity, hypertension, evidence of chronic obstructive pulmonary disease or cyanotic cardiac conditions, and high-altitude living conditions.

SYMPTOMS

- Headaches, weakness, epigastric discomfort, dizziness, sweating, visual disturbances, and plethora
- Pruritus: 50% incidence, can be seen after bathing or water exposure
- Erythromelalgia: burning sensation in toes and fingers
- Palpable splenomegaly: approximately 70%
- Large vessel thrombosis: portal vein, Budd-Chiari
- Thrombosis: 20% initial presenting symptom
- Hemorrhage: 10% major episode
- Thrombocytosis or leukocytosis
- Microcytosis: iron deficiency from rapid red blood cell (RBC) production and iron depletion

Essential Thrombocythemia

- 50% are asymptomatic; diagnosed on routine complete blood (cell) count (CBC) with elevated hemoglobin
- Thrombotic events: more common arterial than venous, such as a myocardial infarction
- Bleeding events: easy bruising, mucosal or gastrointestinal tract bleeding
- Erythromelalgia: burning discomfort in hands and feet
- Splenomegaly
- Recurrent first-trimester spontaneous abortion
- Vasomotor symptoms: light-headedness, headaches, and palpitations

Agnogenic Myeloid Metaplasia

- Anemia in 50%
- Thrombocytosis/leukocytosis
- Constitutional symptoms: fatigue, weight loss, night sweats
- Splenomegaly
- Peripheral smear findings of myelophthisis (also called leuko-erythroblastic): immature cell forms pushed out into circulation as a result of marrow fibrosis and characterized by nucleated RBCs, immature myeloid cells, and teardrop cells
- Increased lactate dehydrogenase (LDH), uric acid (gout symptoms), and alkaline phosphatase
- Extramedullary hematopoiesis in spine

■ Diagnosis

Polycythemia Vera

- A hemoglobin level of more than 17.5 g/dL in men or more than 16.0 g/dL in women is suspicious of PV, and so workup should begin.
- Increased RBC mass was required for the diagnosis but is rarely used today.
- Recheck hemoglobin in 1 month; if still elevated, begin workup.
- If patient has characteristic PV symptoms, begin workup.

Tests for Polycythemia Vera

1. Erythropoietin: If normal or low, consider PV. If high, consider secondary causes (Box 18-1).
2. Bone marrow with cytogenetics: 15% of the time, bone marrow cytogenetics are abnormal.
3. Peripheral blood fluorescence *in situ* hybridization (FISH) for Philadelphia translocation t(9;22), rule out CML.
4. Platelet count of more than 400,000 is often seen.
5. White blood cell (WBC) count more than 12,000/μL.
6. Leukocyte alkaline phosphatase score more than 100.
7. Serum vitamin B_{12} level more than 900.
8. Splenomegaly on examination, order ultrasound of abdomen to evaluate.

■ BOX 18-1 Secondary Causes of Polycythemia

Due to *Increased* Erythropoietin (EPO):
- Pheochromocytoma
- Hemangioblastoma
- Uterine leiomyoma
- Cerebellar hemangioblastoma
- Kidney Lesions: polycystic, hypernephroma, post renal transplant
- Hepatic cysts

Due to Hypoxic Increased EPO:
- Chronic obstructive pulmonary disease
- Cyanotic congenital heart disease with right-to-left shunt
- High-altitude living
- Sleep apnea syndromes
- High oxygen affinity hemoglobin
- Altered hemoglobin oxygen affinity
- Smoking: carboxyhemoglobin

Apparent Polycythemia:
Dehydration
- Diuretic Therapy
- Stress erythrocytosis: smoking, alcohol, hypertension

9. Arterial blood gas analysis.
10. Computed tomographic (CT) scan of abdomen if considering secondary causes.

Tests for Essential Thrombocythemia

- Peripheral smear, to review for abnormality.
- Erythrocyte sedimentation rate (ESR) and C-reactive protein (CRP): If elevated, suspect reactive causes.
- Refer to Box 18-2 for reactive thrombocytosis.
- Complete iron panel: If iron deficient, treat and reassess platelets after iron replete.
- If platelet count is greater than one million, check von Willebrand panel to rule out an acquired von Willebrand disease.
- Peripheral blood FISH for Philadelphia translocation t(9;22), to rule out CML.
- Bone marrow biopsy and aspirate with cytogenetics.

■ BOX 18-2 Reactive Thrombocytosis

Malignant conditions
- Metastatic cancer
- Lymphoma

Nonmalignant hematologic conditions
- Acute blood loss
- Acute hemolytic anemia
- Iron deficiency anemia
- Treatment of vitamin B_{12} deficiency
- Rebound effect after treatment of idiopathic thrombocytopenic purpura
- Rebound effect after ethanol-induced thrombocytopenia

Acute and chronic inflammatory conditions
- Rheumatologic conditions
- Inflammatory bowel disease
- Celiac disease

Tissue damage
- Burns
- Myocardial infarction
- Severe trauma
- Pancreatitis
- Postsplenectomy
- Coronary artery bypass procedures

Infections
Allergic reactions
Exercise
Chronic renal failure

◼ BOX 18-3 Marrow Fibrosis

Myeloid disorders
- Agnogenic myeloid metaplasia
- Chronic myeloid leukemia
- Myelodysplastic syndrome
- Acute leukemia

Non-myeloid disorders
- Metastatic cancer
- Connective tissue disorder
- Infections
- Vitamin D deficiency
- Renal osteodystrophy

Lymphoid disorders
- Hairy cell leukemia
- Multiple myeloma
- Lymphoma

Tests for Agnogenic Myeloid Metaplasia
- Peripheral smear: evaluate for marrow crowding with immature cells on smear.
- Immature cells include early myeloid cells, nucleated RBCs, or teardrop cells.
- Bone marrow biopsy and aspirate with cytogenetics.
- Peripheral blood FISH for Philadelphia translocation t(9;22), to rule out CML.
- Uric acid, LDH, alkaline phosphatase.
- Other causes of marrow fibrosis are listed in Box 18-3

◼ Treatment

Polycythemia Vera
- Phlebotomy: Goal of hematocrit less than 45% in men and less than 42% in women
- Consider aspirin, baby dose = 81 mg, in every patient, unless contraindicated.
- High-risk patients should receive medications along with phlebotomy until hematocrit is lowered into safe range because of high risk of clotting.
- Phosphorous-32 should be avoided because of delayed risk of acute leukemia.
- Interferon is drug of choice during pregnancy.

Essential Thrombocythemia
- Consider aspirin, baby dose = 81 mg, in every patient.

- Low/intermediate risk (age younger than 60 years and no history of thrombosis): controversial; medication to lower platelet count to less than 400,000 or just observe. Recommend lowering platelet count if surgical procedure planned.
- High risk (age older than 60 years or history of thrombosis): medication to lower platelet count to less than 400,000/L.

MEDICATIONS
- Hydroxyurea: Affects all cell lines; side effects include rash, nail changes, cytopenias, and oral or leg ulcers.
- Anagrelide: Affects only platelets; side effects include headache, fluid retention, and congestive heart failure; expensive.
- Interferon-α: Affects all cell lines; side effects include flulike syndrome, depression, and fatigue; drug of choice in pregnancy.
- Aspirin: Contraindicated in acquired von Willebrand disease, history of bleeding, or already on anticoagulation for other comorbidities.
- Aspirin very helpful at relieving erythromelalgia.

Agnogenic Myeloid Metaplasia
- Anemia: Attempt steroids, erythropoietin injections, RBC transfusions as needed.
- Splenectomy: for mechanical or constitutional symptoms, portal hypertension, and severe anemia.
- Allogeneic transplant (from a matched sibling or matched unrelated donor): indicated if younger than 50 years and have a matched sibling, poor chromosomal abnormalities, very poor quality of life with frequent transfusions, or a WBC count more than 30,000/μL and circulating blasts.

■ Prognosis
- Most patients with ET and PV live normal life spans.
- Patients with AMM with normal WBC count and hemoglobin level more than 10 g/dL are expected to have a 10-year life expectancy. Those with a WBC count more than 30,000/μL, hemoglobin level less than 10 g/dL, and/or poor chromosomal abnormalities have a worse survival—in the 2-year range.

Multiple Myeloma

Multiple Myeloma

■ Definitions

Multiple Myeloma
- A malignancy of bone marrow plasma cells, leading to the following:
    1. Disruption of normal marrow function
    2. Damage to surrounding bone
    3. Suppression of normal immune function
    4. Reduced levels of immunoglobulins with increased susceptibility to infection
    5. Impairment of kidney function

Amyloidosis
- Bence Jones light chains cross-link in a beta-pleated fashion and become deposited in organs in the body: kidney, heart, nerves.

Light-Chain Deposition Disease
- Light chains deposit in organs in the body, especially in blood vessels in the eyes and kidneys

Plasmacytomas
- Localized tumors of myeloma cells; can be single or multiple and confined within the bone marrow or in soft tissue

■ Epidemiology

- Estimated new cases: 7800 in women, 6800 in men, total 14,500 cases per year.
- Incidence varies by race; more common in African Americans.
- 8 to 10 per 100,000 population/yr in African Americans.
- 4 per 100,000 population/yr in whites; 1 per 100,000 population/yr in Asians.
- Myeloma comprises 1% of all cancers; it is the second most common blood cancer after lymphomas.
- Trend toward more frequent myeloma in patients younger than 55 years.

■ Pathophysiology

- Multiple myeloma is a malignancy of bone marrow plasma cells.
- Disruption of normal marrow function.
- Damage to surrounding bone.
- Suppression of normal immune function, reduced levels of normal immunoglobulins with increased susceptibility to infection.
- Impairment of kidney function.
- Myeloma cells produce and release a monoclonal protein into the blood and/or urine.
- M protein refers to the monoclonal abnormal protein.
- The monoclonal protein is an immunoglobulin either released in whole or as a light chain or heavy chains only.
- The abnormal monoclonal protein is produced by the aberrant plasma cell and is identified on protein electrophoresis as a monoclonal spike.
- In myeloma, one or more genetic mutations have occurred in the genes responsible for immunoglobulin production; thus, developing an uncontrolled "runaway" plasma cell that is immortal.
- Abnormal structure and function of the immunoglobulin leads to complications:
  1. Abnormally high quantities of the monoclonal protein
  2. Adhere to vessels and clog up the circulation, cause kidney problems, hyperviscosity, nerve damage, predisposition to infection, and bone destruction
  3. Decreased quantity of "normal" immunoglobulins, leading to infections
  4. Excess light chains, called Bence Jones proteins, can freely pass into the urine, causing renal failure

■ Pathologic Manifestations

Blood Findings
- Anemia, leukopenia, thrombocytopenia
- Plasma cell leukemia
- Abnormal clotting
- Circulating monoclonal B lymphocytes
- Reduced immunoglobulins

Skeletal Findings
- Solitary or multiple osteolytic lesions
- Diffuse osteoporosis (osteopenia)

Effects of Bone Destruction
- Hypercalcemia, hypercalciuria
- Bone fractures, vertebral collapse

Plasma Protein Changes
- Hyperproteinemia, hypervolemia
- Monoclonal immunoglobulins (immunoglobulin G [IgG], immunoglobulin D [IgD], immunoglobulin A [IgA], immunoglobulin M [IgM], light chain)
- Narrowed anion gap (low serum sodium concentration)
- Elevated serum β_2-microglobulin level
- Decreased serum albumin level
- Elevated serum interleukin-6 (IL-6) and C-reactive protein levels

Kidney Abnormalities
- Proteinuria
- Tubular dysfunction with acidosis
- Uremia
- Amyloidosis

Extraskeletal Findings
- Soft tissue involvement
- See Table 19-1 for additional definitions

■ Clinical Manifestations
- 70% present with bone pain, lower back or ribs.
- Sudden severe pain can be sign of vertebral collapse.
- Generalized malaise, fatigue from anemia.
- Hypogammaglobulinemia increases the likelihood of infection. Infections noted in myeloma are pneumococcal pneumonia, streptococci, staphylococci, haemophilus, and herpes-zoster infections.
- Hypercalcemia: 30% present with features of a high serum calcium: fatigue, thirst, nausea, deterioration of kidney function.

■ TABLE 19-1 Definitions

Name	Definition
Monoclonal gammopathy of unknown significance (MGUS)	• Monoclonal protein • No pathologic manifestations
Smoldering myeloma	• MGUS, with increasing paraprotein spike

Multiple myeloma	• Bone marrow more than 10% plasma cells or a plasmacytoma and at least *one* of the following:
	    M protein in the serum (usually >3 g/dL)
	    M protein in the urine
	    Lytic bone lesions

- Hyperviscosity: usually with IgM, but can be seen with any elevated paraprotein; can cause easy bruising, nose bleeding, poor vision, headaches, gastrointestinal tract bleeding, and neurologic symptoms. This is more common in Waldenström macroglobulinemia.
- Clotting abnormalities: increased bleeding due to monoclonal proteins binding to clotting factors and platelets. Few patients can form inhibitors to clotting factors, usually factor VIII.
- Neurologic involvement varies; spinal cord compression, polyneuropathies, carpal tunnel syndrome (due to amyloidosis).

■ **Diagnosis**

1. Bone marrow biopsy with cytogenetics and fluorescent *in situ* hybridization (FISH) analysis.
2. Complete blood cell (CBC) count.
3. Chemistry panel with serum albumin.
4. Serum protein electrophoresis (SPEP).
5. Immunofixation: identifies the type of abnormal protein.
6. 24-hour urine protein electrophoresis.
7. Urine protein immunofixation.
8. Metastatic bone survey; plain x-ray films show lytic lesions.
9. Magnetic resonance imaging to focus on particular area if pain or abnormalities identified on bone survey.
10. Nuclear medicine scans: Bone scans are not helpful in lytic bone lesions.
11. Whole-body fluorodeoxyglucose positron emission tomography scans: still being evaluated, sensitive for solitary plasmacytoma and extramedullary disease.
12. After diagnosis established, serum β_2-microglobulin and C-reactive protein can be helpful prognostically.

Staging
- See Table 19-2 for the Durie and Salmon staging.

Types of Monoclonal Protein
SERUM
- IgG (50%)
- IgA (20%)
- IgD (2%)
- IgE (<0.01%)
- IgM, usually classified as Waldenström syndrome (12%)
- Two or more monoclonal spikes (1%)
- Heavy chains only (1%)
- No monoclonal paraprotein, nonsecretory myeloma (3%)

■ TABLE 19-2 Durie and Salmon Staging System

Stage	Criteria
1	All of the following: Hb <10 g/dL Serum calcium normal or <10.5 g/dL Normal bone x-ray findings or solitary plasmacytoma only Low M component: IgG < 5 g/dL, IgA < 3 g/dL Urine light-chain component <4 g/24-hr collection
2	Neither stage 1 nor 3
3	One or more of the following: Hb < 8.5gm/dl Serum calcium >12 mg/dL Advanced lytic bone lesions High M component: IgG < 7 g/dL, IgA > 5 g/dL Urine light-chain M component <12 g/dL

Hb, hemoglobin; IgA, immunoglobulin A; IgG, immunoglobulin G.

■ TABLE 19-3 International Myeloma Staging Prognostic Indicator

Stage	Criteria	Months of Survival Predicted
1	Low β_2-microglobulin < 3.5 mg/dL, albumin >3.0 g/dL	58
2	β_2-Microglobulin < 3.5 mg/dL, but albumin < 3.5 g/dL or β_2-microglobulin = 3.5 to 5.5 mg/dL	42
3	High β_2-microglobulin: >5.5 mg/dL	27

URINE
- Bence Jones, or light chains, types kappa or lambda (11%)

■ **Prognosis** (Table 19-3)

- Age is a separate discriminator. Patients older than 65 years have worse prognostic survival.
- Chromosomal abnormalities: 30% of patients with myeloma have cytogenetic abnormalities.
- Chromosome 3, 5, 7, 9, 11, 15, and 19 trisomies
- Chromosome 13, 14, 16, and 22 monosomies
- Hypodiploidy: poor prognosis
- Hyperdiploidy: favorable prognosis
- Monosomy/deletion chromosome 13: poor prognosis
- Chromosome translocation t(11;14): favorable prognosis

■ Treatment

- There is no cure for myeloma. This must be emphasized to the patient so that realistic goals and expectations can be made regarding treatment.
- Multiple myeloma is treatable and can prolong the life of the patient and improve his or her quality of life through supportive measures.
- The decision to treat is related to the mnemonic **BACK**:
  Bone disease (lytic lesions or osteoporosis)
  Anemia (hemoglobin [Hb] < 10 mg/dL)
  Calcium elevation (>10 mg/dL)
  Kidney dysfunction (creatinine > 2 mg/dL)

Treatment Options

CHEMOTHERAPY

- Melphalan and prednisone: oral treatment that produces excellent remissions in 60% of patients; can damage stem cells and reduce chances of having a successful stem cell transplant subsequently.
- Vincristine, adriamycin, dexamethasone (Decadron) (VAD): excellent remissions in 70% of patients; does not damage stem cells; patients need a central line.
- Various other therapies: dexamethasone alone, cyclophosphamide, combinations of chemotherapy agents.

OTHER OPTIONS

- High-dose chemotherapy with transplant: usually an autologous transplant; this should be considered in all patients younger than 70 years with good performance status.
- Radiation: to specific areas of bone pain or solitary plasmacytomas.
- Maintenance therapy (with steroids).
- Supportive care:
  1. Erythropoietin: to increase Hb
  2. Bisphosphonates: to protect bones and relieve bone pain; to treat hypercalcemia
  3. Antibiotics: as needed for infections
  4. Pain medications: to assist with bone pain
  5. Growth factors: as needed
  6. Brace/corset: to support compression fractures
  7. Physical therapy/exercise
  8. Dialysis/plasmapheresis/surgery: as needed for renal failure, hyperviscosity, and kyphoplasty per orthopedic specialist

NEW TREATMENTS

- Thalidomide and analogue Revimid (antiangiogenesis agents)
- Velcade (proteasome inhibitor)

- Doxil (long-acting adriamycin)
- Trisenox (arsenic trioxide)
- Mini-allo (non-myeloablative) transplant

Waldenström Macroglobulenemia

- Lymphoplasmacytic lymphoma: a cross between a low-grade lymphoma and features of multiple myeloma

■ Epidemiology

- Infrequent disease, 20% as common as multiple myeloma
- Slight male predominance
- Median age 65 years
- More common in whites compared with African Americans

■ Clinical Manifestations

- Hyperviscosity: 30% of individuals present with fatigue, bleeding gums and nose, ocular manifestations (sausage vessels and retinal hemorrhages on examination), neurologic symptoms, stroke.
- Cryoglobulinemia (monoclonal IgM): Raynaud syndrome, palpable purpura, kidney abnormalities.
- Cold agglutinin disease: IgM cold reactive antibodies as red blood cell temperatures approach zero, acrocyanosis/Raynaud syndrome, and episodic hemolysis, which can be very resistant to treatment.
- IgM deposition: in skin or gastrointestinal tract; can cause diarrhea.
- Anemia.
- Increased IgM.
- Depressed uninvolved immunoglobulins and predisposition to infection.
- Hepatosplenomegaly, lymphadenopathy.
- Infiltration of bone marrow.
- Renal manifestations are rare.

■ Diagnostic Evaluation

- IgM > 0.5 g/dL
- More than 25% infiltration of bone marrow with plasma cells and plasmacytoid lymphocytes with characteristic flow cytometry pattern: CD20 positive, CD5 negative, CD10 negative, CD23 negative.
- Special laboratory tests: Cryoglobulins are frequently elevated, and serum hyperviscosity should be evaluated.

■ Treatment

- Waldenström macroglobulinemia is an incurable low-grade lymphoma; thus, treatment should be guided by symptoms.
- Generally, treatment indications are significant anemia, constitutional symptoms, hyperviscosity, significant hepatosplenomegaly or lymphadenopathy, cold agglutinin anemia, cryoglobulinemia, and neuropathy.

Chemotherapy
- Oral chlorambucil
- Fludarabine
- 2-CDA
- Rituxan
- Autologous bone marrow transplant
- Combination chemotherapy

20

Transplantation

Stem Cell Transplant

■ Types of Transplant

- Allogeneic transplant: from one person to another
- Syngeneic transplant: identical twins
- Autologous transplant: use of patient's own previously harvested bone marrow

■ Stem Cell Sources

- Peripheral blood is the preferred choice.
- Peripheral blood tends to more rapidly engraft than bone marrow but has a slightly higher rate of acute and chronic graft-versus-host disease (GVHD).
- Bone marrow harvest is rarely used unless peripheral blood collection is poor.
- Cord blood is rich in stem cells, but not enough stem cells can be harvested, causing slow engraftment.

■ Histocompatibility Testing

- Human leukocyte antigen (HLA-1); A, B, and C are the major loci, expressed on all cells of the body.
- HLA-2DR, HLA-2DQ, and HLA-2DP are the major loci, expressed on B cells and monocytes.
- The major HLA loci are located on chromosome 6 and are closely linked.
- Every individual inherits one chromosome 6 from his or her mother and one from his or her father.
- The chance of any one sibling being a match is one in four.
- A complete match between donor and recipient requires the same alleles at HLA-A, HLA-B, HLA-C, and DR loci.
- The national marrow donor registry has many unrelated transplants, sometimes called matched unrelated donors (MUDs).
- The likelihood of finding a match in an unrelated donor pool is 65% to 70% depending on ethnicity; less success in minority populations.

■ Schema for Transplant Timeline

- Harvest stem cells: The source may be the patient or a sibling.
- High-dose ablative chemotherapy or radiation to destroy tumor cells.
- During bone marrow ablation, the patient has no cells and is at high risk for infection, bleeding, and anemia.
- Transplant stem cells to patient.
- Engraft: Transplant stem cells, regardless of source. Re-populate the marrow and cytopenias resolve.
- In allogeneic stem cell transplants, induction of Graft versus tumor activity
- Nonmyeloablative (mini) transplant: Less intense dosing of chemotherapy; relies heavily on graft-versus-tumor effect.
- Highest time for mortality is the prolonged cytopenias that occur waiting for engraftment.

■ Graft vs. Tumor Effect

- Immunologic differences between donor and host allow the donor cells to attack the host cells. This effect is greatest in acute myeloid leukemia (AML) and chronic myeloid leukemia (CML), but less so in acute lymphocytic leukemia (ALL).

■ Complications

Engraftment

- During period of engraftment, high risk of infections
- Infectious complications: bacterial, fungal (aspergillosis, candida), herpes simplex virus
- Idiopathic pneumonia syndrome during time of neutrophil recovery
- Hepatic veno-occlusive disease: hepatomegaly, jaundice, and ascites
- Hemolytic uremic syndrome/thrombotic thrombocytopenic purpura
- Cardiomyopathy
- Neurologic dysfunction

Acute Graft vs. Host Disease

- Develops within the first 2 months after allogeneic transplant.
- Affects mainly skin, gastrointestinal tract, and liver.
- Treatment: steroids.

Chronic Graft vs. Host Disease

- Late onset, resembles an autoimmune collagen vascular disease.

- Sclerodermatous skin changes, keratoconjunctivitis, sicca syndrome, oral mucosal lesions, esophageal and vaginal strictures, liver disease, and pulmonary insufficiency.
- 30% to 50% develop chronic GVHD.

Long-Term Infectious Complications
- Encapsulated bacteria, *Listeria*, *Salmonella*, *Nocardia*
- Fungal: aspergillosis, PCP
- Viral: respiratory and enteric viruses, cytomegalovirus, varicella zoster, human herpesvirus type 6/7

■ Indications
- AML: poor cytogenetic AML; 40% cure if done during first complete remission, usually allogeneic transplant.
- ALL: useful in Philadelphia-positive t(9;22) ALL; no benefit over chemotherapy in ALL.
- CML: the treatment of choice; controversial with the introduction of Gleevec.
- Chronic lymphocytic leukemia: Autologous and allogeneic transplants have been used in young patients.
- Non-Hodgkin lymphoma: autologous transplant in first relapse after remission obtained with chemotherapy. Also, autologous performed in high-risk patients at initial diagnosis.
- Hodgkin lymphoma: controversial, autologous transplant for relapsed disease.
- Multiple myeloma: autologous transplant done upfront, sometimes tandem, two transplants attempted.
- Breast cancer: controversial, usually indicated because no evidence of superior results over chemotherapy.
- Testicular cancer: controversial, ongoing studies for high-risk and relapsed disease.
- Thalassemia: excellent results.
- Sickle cell disease: trials ongoing.
- Aplastic anemia: recommended in some young high-risk patients.
- Genetic disorders: ongoing trials.

Oncology

Bladder Cancer

■ Epidemiology

- Bladder cancer is the fourth most common cancer in the United States, with 56,500 new cases in 2002.
- Men are more at risk than women, with a 2.5:1.0 male/female ratio.
- The incidence is twice as high in whites as in African Americans.

■ Risk Factors

- Smoking is the most important known risk factor.
- Occupational exposures to arylamines such as in the dye, chemical, and rubber industries have also been implicated.
- Infection with *Schistosoma haematobium* (endemic in Africa, especially the Nile River) increases the risk for squamous cell carcinoma of the bladder.
- Analgesic nephropathy seems to increase the risk, as does hemorrhagic cystitis (as seen with cyclophosphamide use).

■ Pathology

- **Transitional cell carcinoma** is the most common pathology, but adenocarcinoma (6%), squamous cell carcinoma (2%), and small cell carcinoma (<1%) are also found.
- Bladder tumors can be multifocal, which may be due to reimplantation of dislodged tumor cells or to submucosal migration of neoplastic cells.

■ Clinical Manifestations

History

- Most patients present with painless **gross hematuria**.

Diagnostic Evaluation

- Cystoscopy with biopsy is the gold standard; urine cytology is not sensitive but is 100% specific.
- **Intravenous pyelogram** (IVP) is used to evaluate the ureters and kidneys because 2% to 5% of patients will have concomitant or subsequent upper tract tumors, and because it is important to assess ureteral flow and kidney function before treatment.

- There are currently no proven tumor markers, but p53 mutations are commonly found, and p53 overexpression appears to be a poor prognostic marker

■ Staging and Prognosis

- Complete staging can only be accomplished with cystectomy and lymphadenectomy.
- Overall, the 5-year survival is about 80%, but wide stage–based variation exists.
- The American Joint Committee on Cancer (AJCC) TNM staging system and approximate survival rates are summarized in Table 21-1.

■ TABLE 21-1 Summary of Bladder Cancer Staging and Approximate Survival Rates

Stage	T	N	M	5-yr Survival
0	Ta = noninvasive papillary carcinoma Tis = carcinoma *in situ*, confined to the epithelium	N0	M0	75% to 100%
I	T1	N0	M0	60% to 80%
II	T2a = invades superficial muscle T2b = invades deep muscle	N0	M0	40% to 60%
III	T3a = microscopic invasion into perivesical tissue	N0	M0	40% to 60%
III	T3b = macroscopic invasion into perivesical tissue T4a = tumor invades prostate, uterus, or vagina	N0	M0	40% to 60%
IV	T4b = tumor invades pelvic wall or abdominal wall	N0	M0	<30%
	Any T	N0, N1, N2, N3 N1 = single lymph node <2 cm N2 = multiple nodes or one >2 cm, but none >5 cm N3 = any node >5 cm	M0	
	Any T	Any N	M1	

■ Treatment

Ta, T1, Tis (Superficial Tumors)

- Transurethral resection (TUR) plus intravesical therapy (usually bacille Calmette-Guérin [BCG], which is the tuberculosis vaccine).
- For untreated T1 tumors, 50% progress to muscle invasion, so periodic surveillance cystoscopies should be performed; prophylactic radical cystectomy is an alternative.
- About 10% of tumors treated with BCG/TUR progress to muscle-invasive disease.

T2-T4 (Muscle-Invasive Disease)

- Radical cystectomy plus bilateral pelvic lymphadenectomy plus/minus neoadjuvant chemotherapy.
- Clinical trials are investigating bladder-preserving therapies such as TUR plus chemotherapy plus radiation therapy.
- 10-year survival after cystectomy is about 50%.

Metastatic Disease

- The combination methotrexate-vinblastine-adriamycin-cisplatin (MVAC) has been the gold standard for 15 years and offers a 1-year median survival.
- The combination gemcitabine-cisplatin is an acceptable alternative, with a 10-month median survival (ongoing clinical trials are evaluating alternative combinations).

Brain/CNS Cancers

Intracranial Neoplasms

■ Epidemiology

- Primary central nervous system (CNS) tumors affect about 11 per 100,000 Americans yearly.
- Metastatic tumors are more common than primary brain tumors.

■ Risk Factors

- **High-dose ionizing radiation** is the only certain risk factor for primary brain cancers; look for tumors at least a decade after exposure.
- A few genetic syndromes are also associated with brain tumors, namely, Li-Fraumeni cancer syndrome (see Chapter 23), Turcot syndrome (see Chapter 25), tuberous sclerosis, and the neurofibromatoses.
- Other proposed, but unproven, risk factors include cellular telephones, high-tension wires, and exposure to N-nitrosoureas.

■ Pathology

- Tumors can arise from any of the main cellular components of the brain, including the neurons and their supportive cells the glia, as well as the meninges, which overlie the brain and spinal cord.
- Tumors can also arise from intracranial organs such as the pituitary and pineal glands.

Neuronal Tumors

- Gangliocytomas are slow-growing tumors usually found in the third ventricle, hypothalamus, or temporal lobe.
- Medulloblastomas are aggressive tumors of embryonal cell origin occurring usually during childhood and often arising in the cerebellum.
- Cerebral neuroblastomas are very rare tumors of childhood that are similar to peripheral neuroblastomas.

Gliomas

- Gliomas account for more than 60% of intracranial tumors and include the following:

- Astrocytomas
  - Low-grade fibrillary astrocytomas are sometimes difficult to resect because of their size and usually affect young healthy adults.
  - Glioblastoma multiforme accounts for 80% of malignant gliomas; the mean age at diagnosis is 55 years, although some low-grade tumors can transform into this malignant histology ("secondary glioblastoma").
  - Brainstem gliomas comprise 20% of primary CNS tumors in children; these can progress into glioblastomas.
  - Pilocytic astrocytomas are typically benign tumors of childhood; they are usually located in the cerebellum.
- **Oligodendrogliomas** often occur in middle-aged persons and affect hemispheric white matter.
- **Ependymomas** arise from the cells that line the ventricles (ependymal cells, choroid plexus, etc.) or spinal cord and usually affect children and adolescents.

Meningiomas
- Slow-growing, usually benign lesions, more common in adults and with a female preponderance (3:2).
- Other rare tumors include primary pineal malignancies, CNS lymphomas (usually B cell, found especially in patients with acquired immunodeficiency syndrome [AIDS]), pituitary tumors, and germ cell tumors of the CNS.

■ Clinical Manifestations
History
- At least 50% of patients present with headache.
- Seizures occur in more than one fourth of patients with intracranial tumors.
- More rarely, patients will present with focal neurologic signs depending on the size and location of the lesion or the tumor's propensity to bleed.

Diagnostic Evaluation
- **Magnetic resonance imaging** (MRI) of the brain with and without gadolinium is the diagnostic test of choice; if the suspicion is there for an intracranial tumor, this is the first test that should be done.
  - **Low-grade astrocytomas** appear well-circumscribed on MRI (although histologically they are highly infiltrative); they are nonenhancing cerebral lesions without surrounding edema best seen on T2-weighted imaging.
  - **Malignant astrocytomas** reveal ringlike enhancement on MRI scans and do have surrounding edema; glioblastoma multiforme often has central necrosis.

- **Oligodendrogliomas** appear as nonenhancing diffuse white matter lesions best seen on T2-weighted imaging.
- **Meningiomas** are usually skull/bone-based and do not cause edema unless they are high grade.
- **CNS lymphomas** are usually periventricular ring-enhancing lesions.
- **Positron emission tomography** (PET) scanning can be a useful adjunct in that low-grade gliomas tend to underuse glucose, whereas high-grade tumors tend to hypermetabolize.
- **Computed tomography** (CT) scanning can miss low-grade and posterior fossa tumors.
- Most tumors in children are located in the posterior fossa, whereas most intracranial tumors in adults are supratentorial.

■ Staging

- There is no systematic staging system for intracranial neoplasms because most are locally invasive; pathologic grading by the World Health Organization (WHO) system is based on cellular characteristics.

■ Treatment and Prognosis

- **Anticonvulsants** are used in patients who present with seizures; they have not been shown to be useful as prophylaxis in the absence of clinical seizures (except in the perioperative setting).
- **Steroids** (dexamethasone) are useful in the setting of peritumoral edema and mass effect; they should be tapered promptly once treatment is underway.
- **Low-grade and benign tumors** can be resected if significant deficits are not likely postoperatively; such tumors should be resected if they are causing significant neurologic dysfunction.
- **Low-grade astrocytomas** can be treated with radiation when there is evidence of tumor progression; median survival is 5 years. Watch for recurrence with more malignant histology.
- **Malignant astrocytomas** (anaplastic astrocytoma and glioblastoma multiforme) are treated initially with surgical resection when possible, followed by radiation plus/minus chemotherapy with carmustine. Median survival is 1 to 3 years (better when complete resection is possible), and recurrence rates are high.
- **Oligodendrogliomas** have shown good response to chemotherapy with procarbazine, CCNU and vincristine (PCV). Median survival is more than 10 years, although recurrence with more malignant histology is seen (and should be resected).
- **Meningiomas** are slow growing and, if asymptomatic, can simply be observed in older patients; smaller ones can be removed if technically feasible. Recurrence is common and radiation can slow regrowth.

■ **Epidemiology**

- Women older than 50 years (5% are younger than 40 years).
- Second most common cancer diagnosed in American women.
- More common in the United States than in the Eastern Hemisphere.
- One in eight to nine American women will develop breast cancer in her lifetime.

■ **Risk Factors**

- Factors known to increase risk include previous diagnosis with breast cancer or ductal carcinoma *in situ* (DCIS) or lobular carcinoma *in situ* (LCIS) or atypical hyperplasia, nulliparity, late parity (first pregnancy after age 35 years), young age at menarche.
- Germline mutations in the **BRCA1** and **BRCA2** genes account for fewer than 10% of all breast cancers; however, the risk in individuals with these mutations is extremely high (35% to 70% cumulative risk up to age 60 years), and such women are given the option of prophylactic mastectomy plus/minus selective estrogen receptor modulators.
- Factors thought to increase risk but still controversial are smoking, inactivity/obesity during adolescence and young adulthood, hormone replacement therapy, and significant daily alcohol consumption.
- Primary prevention strategies proven to reduce mortality include annual mammography between ages 50 and 69 years; mammography before age 50 years in women without risk factors is often done, though not proven to change mortality.
- Self-breast examination and even clinical breast examination are not proven to reduce mortality.

■ **Pathology**

Fibroadenomas

- The most common benign breast tumors; usually located in the upper outer quadrant, they are well circumscribed and movable.
- Consist of both fibrous and glandular cells.

- Hormonal influences such as menses and pregnancy may influence size.

Phyllodes Tumors
- Arise from intralobular stroma of the breast and are usually benign.
- Cystosarcoma phyllodes is a malignant version that can behave more aggressively.

Intraductal Papillomas
- Arise from within ducts usually close to the nipple and are usually benign.
- They do often recur, and when they exist in groups, there is an increased risk of malignant transformation (papillocarcinoma).

Ductal Carcinoma In Situ
- DCIS consists of malignant cells that do not invade the basement membrane of breast ducts.
- Of the five histologic subtypes, **comedocarcinoma** is considered high grade and predictive of recurrence.

Lobular Carcinoma In Situ
- LCIS is characterized by a benign-appearing proliferation of terminal ducts and ductules that is often multifocal and bilateral.
- In untreated patients, more than 30% will develop invasive infiltrating ductal or lobular carcinoma in the affected or contralateral breast.

Infiltrating Ductal Carcinoma
- The most common breast cancer histology, accounting for about 75% of breast cancers.
- **Scirrhous** carcinoma is the most common subtype and is characterized by well-demarcated hard nodules consisting of cords and nests of malignant ductal cells.
- **Medullary** carcinoma is much less common and characterized by a lymphocytic infiltrate; these tumors have a better prognosis.
- **Mucinous** carcinoma is a more slow-growing subtype, often diagnosed in elderly women and on resection exhibits a gelatinous consistency.
- **Paget disease** is a subtype in which malignant ductal cells extend intraepithelially to the skin of the nipple.

Invasive Lobular Carcinoma
- Invasive lobular carcinoma constitutes only about 10% of breast cancers and like its noninvasive counterpart arises from terminal ductules of breast lobules.

- Tumor cells are often arranged in single files/strands, but at times it may be difficult to distinguish from ductal carcinomas.
- Many are multicentric within a breast and about 20% are bilateral.

Clinical Manifestations

History

- About 65% of patients will present with a breast lump.
- More patients are presenting with asymptomatic screening mammography abnormalities.
- Any complaints of skin changes overlying the breast or nipple, as well as nipple discharge, should be further evaluated (see later discussion).
- A full family history is very important and should include other cancer types.

Diagnostic Evaluation

- The diagnostic approach to a breast mass should start with the physical examination noting skin changes, nipple discharge, and adenopathy in the axillae and supraclavicular regions.
- The "triple screen" employs mammography, ultrasound, and fine needle aspiration (FNA) for further evaluation.
- If suspicion is high for the diagnosis of breast cancer and the patient is asymptomatic, relevant laboratories include liver studies with calcium and alkaline phosphatase to assess for liver and bony metastases, as well as a complete blood cell (CBC) count to assess for anemia and superimposing infection.
- Computed tomography (CT) scanning of the chest, abdomen, and pelvis and/or PET scan is used to evaluate for metastases if the patient is symptomatic or if the laboratory results are abnormal.
- Mammography is recommended in the contralateral breast before surgical intervention.
- MRI is particularly helpful in screening lobular carcinoma and BRCA1/2 carriers.
- If there is nothing to suggest distant metastases, the surgeons will resect the lesion with margins and perform a **sentinel node biopsy,** in which blue dye is injected into the tumor area; the first node to pick up the dye is resected and examined for malignant cells. The test has a 95% negative predictive value; that is, if no malignant cells are noted, the surgeons finish resection of the mass and do no further nodal removal.
- If the sentinel node biopsy is positive, or if there is evidence of stage III or greater disease, a formal axillary nodal dissection (removal of 10 to 15 nodes is performed).
- Many surgeons now routinely perform sentinel node biopsies even for DCIS.

■ Staging/Prognosis

- The American Joint Committee on Cancer TNM staging system is the most widely used for breast cancer.
- Survival in breast cancer appears to be inversely correlated to the number of axillary nodal metastases present.
- Relapse appears to be related to the number of nodal metastases as well.
- A summary of the staging system and approximate survival rates is outlined in Table 23-1.

■ Treatment

- **Breast-conserving therapy** has been proven safe and effective for DCIS and stage I/II tumors (<4 cm); sentinel lymph node biopsy is usually pursued to confirm localized disease.
  - Postoperative breast radiation (not to the nodes) is standard of care; it has been shown to reduce recurrence

■ TABLE 23-1 AJCC TNM Staging System for Breast Cancer

Stage	Description	Survival Rate
Stage I	Tumor ≤2 cm, no nodes	98% 5-yr survival
Stage IIA	One to three axillary nodes without primary breast tumor, or tumor ≤2 cm with one to three axillary lymph nodes, or tumor ≤2 cm with microscopic invasion of internal mammary node(s) by sentinel lymph node biopsy, or tumor 2 to 5 cm without nodal involvement	88% 5-yr survival
Stage IIB	Tumor 2 to 5 cm with one to three axillary nodes, or tumor >5 cm without extension into other organs or lymph nodes	76% 5-yr survival
Stage IIIA	No primary breast tumor but four to nine axillary lymph nodes affected, or tumor up to 5 cm with four to nine axillary nodes, or tumor >5 cm with up to nine axillary nodes or with macroscopic involvement of internal mammary node(s) (by examination or imaging)	56% 5-yr survival
Stage IIIB	Tumor of any size with direct extension into the skin or chest wall with/without nodes, or any tumor size with more than ten axillary lymph nodes or ipsilateral supraclavicular/ infraclavicular lymph node involvement	49% 5-yr survival
Stage IV	Distant metastases, including contralateral lymph node spread	16% 5-yr survival

- Chemotherapy is not usually given for tumors smaller than 1 cm with negative nodes.
- Adjuvant chemotherapy is recommended for tumors larger than 2 cm, tumors between 1-2 cms with unfavorable prognostic markers and in lymph node-positive patients.
- Hormonal manipulation is suggested in estrogen receptor + (ER+), progesterone receptor + (PR+) tumors. Tamoxifen is offered to pre-menopausal women. An aromatase inhibitor is offered to post-menopausal women. There are three known aromatase inhibitors: Anastrazole (Arimidex), Letrozole (Femara), and Exemestane (Aromasin).
- Mastectomy is suggested for tumors larger than 4 to 5 cm, followed by chemotherapy plus/minus x-radiation therapy.
- Radiation is given to tumors larger than 5 cm and to women with more than four lymph nodes positive with cancer. Ongoing studies are accessing the benefit of radiation for local control in patients with less than four nodes positive.
- Neoadjuvant (preoperative) chemotherapy is recommended for patients with localized Stage III disease as an attempt to downstage tumors for surgical resection. There is a trend towards neoadjuvant chemotherapy in earlier stage disease in order to skrink the tumor for lumpectomy and to assess in vivo responsiveness to chemotherapy. This has not shown a survival advantage over adjuvant chemotherapy.
- Metastatic disease (Stage IV) is treated with many different modalities. It is **not** curable.
- Hormonal manipulation is preferred for ER+, PR+ disease not in visceral crisis.
  - Tamoxifen or aromatase inhibitors are considered.
  - Second line manipulations include switching to another aromatase inhibitor, Fulvestrant (Faslodex), or Progesterone (Megace).
- Chemotherapy is the only option in ER−, PR− disease. Usually single agent chemotherapy is the standard with various agents depending on the adjuvant chemotherapy given. Examples are Navelbine, Taxanes, Gemzar, Carboplantinum, and the pill Xeloda. Combination chemotherapy is given for visceral crises; for rapid control of tumor bulk.
- Her-2/neu disease represents a disease that is responsive to Herceptin, a monoclonal antibody directed against the Her-2/neu gene. Herceptin can be given in any stage and setting and is synergistic with many different chemotherapy agents.

Cervical Cancer

Epidemiology

- Both the incidence of and death rates from cervical cancer have decreased dramatically in developed countries where regular Pap smears are part of routine health care for women.
- The incidence is highest in Vietnamese women, followed by Hispanic, native Alaskan, Korean, and African American women.
- The lowest incidence is in Japanese women.
- Tragically, in some developing countries, cervical cancer is still the leading cause of death in women.
- Peak incidence occurs during the fourth decade of life.

Risk Factors

- Multiple sexual partners and early age at first intercourse are associated with higher risk (perhaps because of more likely exposure to human papillomavirus [HPV]).
- **HPV,** especially subtypes 16, 18, 31, 33, 35, and 45, are associated with higher risk for cancer (6, 11, 42, and 44 are low-risk subtypes).
  - Worldwide HPV infection rates are significantly higher than cervical cancer rates, suggesting that other factors must contribute to pathogenesis.
  - HPV DNA is found in about 85% of cervical cancers.
- **Human immunodeficiency virus** (HIV) is an important cofactor for HPV, significantly increasing the risk for higher grade lesions and neoplasia; cervical cancer is now an acquired immunodeficiency syndrome (AIDS)–defining condition.

Pathology

- **Squamous cell carcinoma** constitutes about 80% of cervical cancers, with adenocarcinoma accounting for most of the remainder; rarely, sarcomas, lymphomas, and melanomas are found.
- The transformation of normal cells to precancerous and cancerous lesions tends to occur at the **squamocolumnar junction,** where the normal squamous cells of the vagina meet the columnar cells of the uterine cervix.

- **Precancerous lesions** may be reported in the following ways, depending on the system used by the pathologist reading the Pap smear:
  - Mild dysplasia may be referred to as low-grade squamous intraepithelial lesion (LGSIL) or cervical intraepithelial neoplasia (CIN I).
  - Moderate to severe dysplasia may be referred to as high-grade squamous intraepithelial lesion (HGSIL) or CIN II to CIN III or carcinoma *in situ* (CIS).
  - ASCUS means atypical squamous cells of unknown significance and essentially calls for repeated Pap smears and HPV testing.

■ Clinical Manifestations

History

- Precancerous lesions are usually asymptomatic; cancerous lesions may be asymptomatic as well or they may present with menometrorrhagia (bleeding between periods), postcoital bleeding, or dyspareunia (pain with intercourse).
- A thorough history should document sexual risk factors and risk factors for HIV and the results of previous Pap smears.

Diagnostic Evaluation

- Yearly Pap screening is recommended for all adult or sexually active women.
- If the Pap smear is abnormal, colposcopy allows for a magnified view of the cervical lining.
- Biopsy is usually performed via loop electrosurgical excision (LEEP).
- Computed tomography (CT) or magnetic resonance imaging (MRI) of the pelvis is used to determine the extent of involvement of pelvic structures and lymph nodes; chest x-ray (CXR) is usually performed to rule out distant metastases.
- Intravenous pyelogram and barium enema are usually not necessary when CT or MRI are available; however, with advanced disease cystoscopy may be pursued to identify bladder invasion.

■ Staging

- As with uterine cancer, the staging system for cervical cancer comes from the International Federation of Gynecology and Obstetrics (FIGO).
- Stage I tumors involve only the cervix; 5-year survival ranges from 85% to 100%.
- Stage II tumors may extend to the upper two thirds of the vagina; 5-year survival is about 85% to 90%.

- Stage III tumors may involve the pelvic wall or the lower one third of the vagina; 5-year survival is around 50%.
- Stage IV tumors extend beyond the pelvic wall and may involve the bladder mucosa, the rectum, or distant organs; 5-year survival is usually less than 10%.

■ Treatment

- Simple or radical hysterectomy are performed for stage I/II tumors, with postoperative radiation for patients at high risk of recurrence (larger lesions).
- For lesions larger than 4 cm, chemoradiation may be the initial therapy.
- Neoadjuvant (preoperative) chemotherapy has not been shown to improve survival.
- For advanced disease, monotherapy option include cisplatin, ifosfamide, the taxanes, or irinotecan.
- Studies evaluating combination chemotherapy suggest that response rates are better than those for monotherapy.

Colorectal and Anal Cancers

■ Epidemiology

- Colorectal and anal cancers are the second leading cause of cancer death in the United States, although mortality rates are decreasing as better screening leads to earlier diagnosis.
- The leading cancer diagnosed in Americans older than 75 years.
- Although the incidence is highest in industrialized nations, one third of colorectal cancers are diagnosed in the developing world.
- Slightly more common in men than women.
- Most colorectal cancers arise from dysplastic polyps.
- Anal canal cancers are more common in women and usually in people older than 60 years.

■ Risk Factors

- Increased physical activity has been inversely correlated to colon cancer in both men and women.
- Use of hormone replacement therapy, particularly if used for longer than 5 years, may reduce the risk of colorectal malignancy.
- High daily intake of red meat and processed meat has been associated with increased incidence of colorectal cancers.
- Tobacco likely increases the risk.
- Receptive anal intercourse appears to increase the risk for anal cancers.
- The genetic syndromes associated with colorectal cancer are outlined in Box 25-1.
- **Hamartomas** are benign mucosal lesions without malignant potential; however, adenomas may occur in their midst, thus requiring surveillance.
  - **Juvenile polyposis syndrome** is an autosomal dominant disorder in which children (usually younger than 5 years) exhibit large hamartomatous polyps, often in the rectum.
  - **Peutz-Jeghers syndrome** is another rare autosomal dominant disorder characterized by mucocutaneous pigmented lesions and hamartomas anywhere along the gastrointestinal (GI) tract, especially the small bowel; there is an increased risk of

■ BOX 25-1 Genetic Syndromes Associated with Colorectal Cancer

Hereditary nonpolyposis colorectal cancer (HNPCC) (Lynch syndrome)
- Accounts for only 1% to 3% of colorectal cancers.
- Three or more first-degree relatives, spanning two generations, at least one diagnosed before age 50 years (these "Amsterdam criteria" may be too exclusive).
- Median age at diagnosis, 45 years.
- Few "flat" lesions, often in the right colon.
- Lesions become cancerous rapidly requiring frequent colonoscopy (every 2 years).
- Multiple mutation types, most often in MLH1 and MSH2, DNA repair genes.
- Type II HNPCC involves extracolonic tumors, especially uterine, biliary, urinary, and small intestine ("Turcot syndrome" involves brain tumors, "Muir-Torre syndrome" involves skin tumors).

Familial adenomatous polyposis (FAP)
- Autosomal dominant defect in the APC (adenomatous polyposis coli) gene, which is a tumor suppressor gene, chromosome 5.
- More than 100, and as many as 2500, polyps develop in the colonic mucosa by adolescence.
- Histology usually tubular adenomas.
- Malignant transformation occurs more than 10 to 15 years from the onset of adenomas in 100% of cases!
- Often associated with malignancy in the left colon.
- Gardner syndrome is a subset of FAP, which in addition to the intestinal polyps, involves multiple osteomas (skull, mandible, long bones).
- Colonoscopy should begin during adolescence in affected families, and prophylactic colectomy is advised

pancreatic, breast, lung, uterine, and ovarian carcinomas with this syndrome.
- The inflammatory bowel diseases both increase the risk of colorectal cancer; ulcerative colitis increases it by about fivefold more than Crohn disease.
  - Screening colonoscopy should begin 8 years after pancolitis diagnosed (by baseline diagnostic colonoscopy) and repeated every 1 to 2 years; prophylactic colectomy is recommended once dysplasia is detected.
- New data suggest that aspirin, nonsteroidal antiinflammatory drugs (NSAIDS), and cyclooxygenase-2 (COX-2) inhibitors may prevent malignant transformation of polyps in high-risk patients.

■ Pathology

- More than 95% of large intestinal malignancies are adenocarcinomas.
- About 25% are right-sided lesions; 50% are left sided.

- **Right-sided lesions** tend to grow lengthwise along the cecum/ascending colon.
- **Left-sided lesions** are classically "napkin-ring" or "apple-core," meaning that they encircle and constrict a region of bowel.
- Other malignant histologies include squamous cell carcinomas (especially in the distal rectum), carcinoid tumors, small cell carcinomas, adenosquamous and undifferentiated carcinomas, and lymphomas (these last mostly in the anal canal).
- Most anal canal malignancies are squamous cell carcinomas.

■ Clinical Manifestations

History
- As discussed in the heme section, microcytic anemia in a male older than 50 years or a postmenopausal woman is a sign of GI tract malignancy until proven otherwise.
- Fatigue, anemia, and weight loss are nonspecific complaints that should prompt investigation of the GI tract; these are more common with right colonic lesions.
- Changes in bowel habits, such as thin-caliber stools, melena, crampy abdominal pain, constipation, or diarrhea, also warrant investigation with colonoscopy in older persons; these tend to signify left colonic lesions.
- Tenesmus (sense of incomplete emptying of stool), rectal bleeding, or pain on defecation are more classic for rectal cancer.

Diagnostic Evaluation
- In symptomatic patients, a thorough family history should be elicited; digital rectal examination is an important part of the physical examination.
- **Fecal occult blood** testing is used as a screening test; if the index of suspicion is sufficiently high or an occult blood test result is positive, a colonoscopy should be performed.
- **Colonoscopy** is the gold standard because suspicious lesions can be biopsied.
- **Double-contrast barium enema** can be performed for lower risk patients; however, beware of a relatively high false-negative rate.

■ Staging and Prognosis
- The TNM staging system is outlined in Table 25-1.

■ Treatment
- Surgery is the mainstay for localized disease (Table 25-2).
- For stage II and III rectal carcinomas, postoperative chemoradiation is the standard of care.
- Resection of hepatic metastases is often done now for otherwise localized colorectal tumors and can be curative.

■ TABLE 25-1 Summary of the TNM Colorectal Staging System and Approximate Survival Rates

Stage	Description	Survival Rate
Stage I	Tumor limited to submucosa or muscularis propria; no nodes	90% 5-yr survival
Stage II	Tumor invades the through the muscularis into the subserosa or pericolic/perirectal tissue; or tumor invades the visceral peritoneum or local structures; no nodes	70% 5-yr survival
Stage III	Any tumor with metastases in perirectal or pericolic lymph nodes	45% 5-yr survival
Stage IV	Distant metastases	<5% 5-yr survival

■ TABLE 25-2 Overview of Stage-Based Approach to Treatment of Colorectal Tumors

Stage	Treatment
Stage I disease	Surgical resection
Stage II disease	Surgical resection; adjuvant chemotherapy confers a very small 2-3% survival benefit in some studies, usually with a continuous infusion 5-FU/LV based regiment (FOLFOX). This is controversial.
Stage III disease	Surgical resection; adjuvant chemotherapy with a 5-FU/LV based regiment and Oxaliplatin (FOLFOX), standard of care.
Stage IV/advanced Stage III	5-FU-LV continuous based regiments with Oxaliplatin (FOLFOX) or Irinotecan (IFL) and Avastin (VEGF inhibitor). Capecitabine pills and Cetuximab with or without Irinotecan are other second line options. Capecitabine pills may replace continuous infusion 5-FU; ongoing studies are pending.

• For anal cancer, local excision is performed for very small superficial lesions, but chemoradiation is the standard of care for most of these patients (with abdominoperineal resection for patients whose biopsies are still positive).

26

Esophageal Cancer

■ Epidemiology

- The incidence is increasing; about 14,000 new cases per year in the United States.
- 3:1 male/female ratio.
- Highest incidence in African American men.
- Mean age at diagnosis is 67 years.
- Adenocarcinoma is overtaking squamous cell carcinoma as the most common histologic type.

■ Risk Factors

- Smoking is a risk factor for both squamous cell and adenocarcinoma of the esophagus.
- Whereas squamous cell cancer risk decreases substantially about 10 years after cessation, the risk for adenocarcinoma does not seem to decline with cessation.
- Mediastinal radiation for previous malignancies (e.g., breast cancer, lymphoma) is also a risk factor for both squamous cell and adenocarcinoma of the esophagus.
- Alcohol use, particularly when combined with tobacco smoking, is a known risk factor for squamous cell carcinomas.
- Chronic chemical irritation to the esophagus can also predispose to squamous cell carcinoma; for example, achalasia, lye ingestion, esophageal diverticula, and frequent consumption of extremely hot fluids.
- An autosomal dominant disorder known as tylosis and characterized by hyperkeratosis of the palms and soles is the only known genetic abnormality associated with esophageal squamous cell carcinoma; affected persons have up to 95% risk of developing cancer by age 70 years.
- Gastroesophageal reflux disease can promote Barrett esophagus, which has an annual rate of transformation to adenocarcinoma of 0.5%.

■ Pathology

- Adenocarcinomas and squamous cell carcinomas constitute most esophageal neoplasms; rarely, carcinoids, melanomas, and sarcomas are diagnosed in this organ.

- Squamous cell carcinomas occur predominantly in the middle and lower thirds of the esophagus; about 20% are located in the upper third.
- Squamous cell tumors spread locally through the wall of the esophagus and into mediastinal structures and lymph nodes.
- Adenocarcinomas tend to occur in the distal esophagus; these glandular cells are easily recognized among the normal squamous epithelium of the esophagus.
- Adenocarcinomas also spread locally through the esophageal wall and sometimes into the gastric cardia.

■ Clinical Manifestations

History

- Onset is usually insidious, but most patients ultimately admit to dysphagia, first to solids and progressing to liquids, with consequent weight loss.
- Aspiration of food is a particularly bad sign, which may indicate tracheoesophageal fistula.

Diagnostic Evaluation

- Patients with dysphagia or odynophagia in the outpatient setting should first be evaluated with a barium swallow examination.
- Biopsy can be obtained via endoscopy.
- Once the diagnosis is made, computed tomography scanning of the chest, abdomen, and pelvis should be pursued to rule out metastatic disease.
- Endoscopic ultrasound is useful in localized disease to determine the depth of involvement.
- Positron emission tomography scanning is increasingly becoming the modality of choice for ruling out metastases and lymph node involvement.

■ Staging and Prognosis

- Unfortunately, esophageal cancers are often detected in later stages and have poor overall 5-year survival rates of about 15%. The TNM staging system and approximate survival rates are summarized in Table 26-1.

■ Treatment

- Surgery remains the mainstay of therapy for patients with localized disease (stages I through III).

■ TABLE 26-1 Esophageal Cancer Staging and Approximate Survival Rates

Stage	Description	Survival Rate
Stage I	Confined to *submucosa/lamina propria*	75% 5-yr survival
Stage IIA	Invades the *muscularis propria or adventitia*	35% 5-yr survival
Stage IIB	Invades the lamina or muscularis and *regional lymph nodes*	20% 5-yr survival
Stage III	Invades the *adventitia and regional nodes,* or invades *local structures* plus/minus regional nodes	12% 5-yr survival
Stage IVA	Invades celiac or cervical nodes	<5% 5-yr survival
Stage IVB	*Distant metastases*	<1% 1-yr survival

- Despite few data supporting improved survival with preoperative chemotherapy and radiation, many centers still offer the combination.
- No survival advantage has been shown for postoperative chemotherapy/radiation.
- For nonsurgical candidates, radiation combined with chemotherapy (cisplatin-fluorouracil, usually) has led to survival rates almost comparable to those for surgery.

Gastric Cancer

■ **Epidemiology**

- The incidence of gastric cancer is particularly high in Japan and Korea and in developing countries where gastric infection with *Helicobacter pylori* is endemic.
- The male/female ratio is about 2:1.
- The mean age at diagnosis is 62 years.
- Although there has been an overall decline in gastric cancer among Western countries, there has been a marked increase in cancers of the proximal stomach (cardia); these neoplasms are not related to *H. pylori* infection.

■ **Risk Factors**

- The genetic risk factors include type A blood (weak association), pernicious anemia, family history, hereditary nonpolyposis coli, and Li-Fraumeni syndrome.
- The modifiable risk factors include a high salt and nitrate intake (salted, pickled, chemically preserved foods), low vitamin A/C intake from fresh fruits and vegetables, cigarette smoking, *H. pylori* infection, and radiation exposure.

■ **Pathology**

- 90% of gastric neoplasms are carcinomas, which are further characterized as intestinal or diffuse type.

Intestinal Type

- Composed of neoplastic glands similar to those found in the intestinal mucosa, this type of neoplasm follows a typical pattern of progression from gastritis to atrophy to intestinal metaplasia to dysplasia to carcinoma.
- Associated with *H. pylori*.
- Decreasing incidence.
- Spreads locally.

Diffuse Variant

- Composed of gastric cells whose neoplastic nuclei push their cytoplasm to the periphery ("signet ring" cells), this tumor has

an infiltrative growth pattern, which may cause fibrosis of the stomach wall.
- More proximally located, usually in the cardia.
- Increasing incidence.
- Early hematogenous spread.

Classic Sites of Metastases
- Virchow node (left supraclavicular node)
- Krukenberg tumor (mets to ovaries)
- Sister Mary Joseph node (umbilical lymph node representing peritoneal mets)
- Blumer shelf (palpable as a hard shelf between the vagina and rectum on digital examination)

Other Tumors of the Stomach
- These include lymphomas (5%), carcinoids (3%), and malignant spindle cell tumors (2%)
- Primary stomach lymphomas (also known as mucosa-associated lymphoid tumors [MALT]) have been shown to regress with successful eradication of *H. pylori* infection.

■ Clinical Manifestations

History
- Patients classically present with epigastric discomfort, melena, weight loss, nausea, and/or vomiting.

Diagnostic Evaluation
- Workup usually begins with a double-contrast radiographic study ("barium swallow" or upper gastrointestinal [GI] series); a definitive diagnosis is made by *endoscopic biopsy*.

■ Staging

The standard American Joint Committee Cancer (AJCC) TNM system is used (Box 27-1). Tumor characteristics are assessed by biopsy and by endoscopic ultrasound for tumor depth (where available). Nodal status and presence of metastases are best evaluated with computed tomography (CT) scanning. Definitive assessment of nodes is achieved surgically (once the tumor is deemed resectable); at least 15 nodes must be removed for adequate staging.

■ Treatment and Prognosis

- Early diagnosis is key. The Japanese tend to detect gastric cancer at earlier stages than Americans because of more aggressive screening.
- Worldwide, surgery remains the cornerstone of curative therapy and is often pursued for palliation as well.

■ **BOX 27-1 TNM Characteristics and Staging of Gastric Cancer**

T: Tumor characteristics

Tis	Carcinoma *in situ*
T1	Mucosa/submucosal invasion
T2	Muscularis invasion
T3	Serosal invasion
T4	Adjacent organ

N: Nodal status

N0	All nodes negative
N1	1–6 positive nodes
N2	7–15 positive nodes
N3	≥16 nodes

M: metastases

M0	No mets
M1	Any distant metastases = stage IV disease

Overall gastric cancer staging

Stage	0	Tis
Stage	1A	T1 N0 M0
	1B	T1 N1, T2 N0, M0
Stage	II	T1 N2, T2 N1, T3 N0
Stage	IIIA	T2 N2, T3 N1, T4 N0
Stage	IIIB	T3 N2, T4 N1, M0
Stage	IV	T4 N2, *any M1*

- Generally, total gastrectomy is performed; subtotal gastrectomy can be done for smaller tumors of the antrum or distal body.
- The extent of lymphadenectomy remains controversial; a D1 resection involves only the perigastric nodes, whereas D2 through D4 resections, preferred by Japanese surgeons, involve en bloc resection of more distal lymph node groups (e.g., hepatic, periaortic, and pancreatic/splenic).

Adjuvant/Neoadjuvant Chemoradiation

- Chemotherapy is indicated for patients with stage III and IV disease and seems to have benefit for palliation and for prolonging survival; downstaging can make these patients eligible for surgery.
- Cisplatin and 5-fluorouracil are commonly used for gastric cancer. Epirubicin, taxanes, and irinotecan are other options.
- Chemoradiation is given after curative resection to prevent recurrence.
- Irinotecan is a new agent that appears promising.

■ TABLE 27-1 Approximate Survival Rates in Gastric Cancer	
Stage	Survival Rate
Stage I	85%
Stage II	55%
Stage III	10%
Stage IV	3%

■ **Survival**

- Approximate 5-year survivals are listed in Table 27-1.
- Median survival for stage IV disease is about 7 months (less without chemotherapy and can be longer with palliative surgery).

Head and Neck Cancers

■ Epidemiology

- Head and neck cancers include nasopharyngeal, laryngeal, and oral cavity cancers, which are relatively uncommon.
- The male/female ratio is approximately 3:1.
- Onset is usually in the fifth to sixth decade of life.
- There is no racial predominance, but the incidence appears to be increasing in African American men.

■ Risk Factors

- Tobacco use clearly increases the risk of both primary and second primary head and neck cancers.
- Cigar smoking and tobacco chewing both increase the risk of head and neck tumors, especially of the oral cavity.
- Alcohol use, especially when combined with tobacco use, increases the risk.
- Infection with Epstein-Barr virus (EBV) has been associated with the high rate of nasopharyngeal cancer in Asia and North Africa; there may be some interaction also with high intake of salted meat and fish.
- Betel nut chewing or tobacco chewing is thought to be associated with the higher rates of laryngeal cancer in India and other parts of Asia.
- Sun exposure predisposes to cancers of the lip.

■ Pathology

- More than 95% of cancers of the oral cavity and larynx are squamous cell carcinomas; other types include salivary gland adenocarcinomas, melanomas, neuroendocrine tumors, and lymphomas.
- **Nasopharyngeal carcinomas** are also usually squamous cell; EBV has been detected in the epithelial cells of a large proportion of these tumors (its exact role in oncogenesis in this area is unclear).
- The most common tumor of the parotid gland is the **pleomorphic adenoma**, which is benign; the most common malignant salivary gland tumor, also usually in the parotid gland, is the **mucoepidermoid carcinoma**.

- Tumors of the pinna of the ear are usually related to sun exposure and include basal cell and squamous cell carcinoma; tumors of the external ear canal are usually squamous cell and unrelated to sun exposure.

■ Clinical Manifestations

History

- Index of suspicion may be raised by alcohol/tobacco use in asymptomatic patients.
- Any patient with complaints of voice change, masses, mucosal lesions or "bumps," odynophagia (pain on swallowing), halitosis, or epistaxis should be evaluated to rule out malignancy if these do not resolve in a few weeks.

Diagnostic Evaluation

- A full HEENT examination includes palpation with a gloved finger of the floor of the mouth, salivary glands, tongue, and gums, as well as inspection of the ear and nasal canals.
- **Leukoplakia** is a white plaque that does not scrape off; although it can have various causes, malignancy should be ruled out.
- **Erythroplakia** is a red velvety lesion in the oropharynx that is even more concerning for malignancy.
- A more formal evaluation by the ear, nose, and throat (ENT) team should be pursued and consists of the following:
  - **Indirect laryngoscopy** in which a mirror is used to evaluate the nasopharynx, hypopharynx, and larynx including the vocal cords
  - **Direct laryngoscopy** in which a camera is passed through the nasal canal to more thoroughly inspect the same regions
  - **"Triple endoscopy"** should be performed in any patient with a head and neck cancer to rule out a second primary; this consists of endoscopy, direct laryngoscopy, and bronchoscopy
- Computed tomography (CT) scanning is the imaging study of choice for head and neck tumors, although in some cases magnetic resonance imaging is more helpful in precisely delineating tumor extent.
- Fine needle aspiration rather than core biopsy should be the initial maneuver to obtain tissue.
- Chest x-ray should be performed to rule out a second lung primary; this should be done on a yearly basis even after definitive therapy, because head and neck tumors are associated with an increased risk of later development of lung cancer.
- Laboratories are not typically useful, although EBV markers may be drawn in the setting of nasopharyngeal tumors.

■ Staging

- The TNM staging system is used, with stages I and II representing localized disease and stages III and IV representing invasive disease and lymph node involvement.

■ Treatment and Prognosis

- Stage I and II disease is treated with surgery or radiation with concomitant chemotherapy, depending on the anatomic location.
- Postoperative radiation reduces recurrence.
- Combination chemotherapy is often used for stages III and IV disease, but the effect on overall survival may not be significant.
- In general, 5-year survival for stage I/II disease is 80%, and for stage III/IV disease, it is less than 40%.
- Vitamin A or its analogues (retinoids) may be effective chemoprevention against primary and/or second primary head and neck tumors.

29 Hepatocellular Carcinoma

■ Epidemiology

- The incidence of hepatocellular carcinoma (HCC) is highest in China, Southeast Asia, and sub-Saharan Africa where chronic hepatitis B virus (HBV) is endemic.
- The incidence is lowest in developed regions such as the United States and Europe.
- HCC is almost three times as common in men than women.
- In the United States, blacks are affected more commonly than whites.

■ Risk Factors

- Chronic HBV and HCV remain the most important risk factors.
- Chronic liver diseases such as hemochromatosis, α_1-antitrypsin deficiency, and alcoholism also predispose to HCC.
- **Aflatoxin B**, a product of the mold *Aspergillus flavus*, is found in poorly stored food products (e.g., nuts) in developing countries and is associated with HCC.
- About 70% of patients with HCC have underlying cirrhosis.

■ Pathology

- More than 90% of primary liver neoplasms are hepatocellular carcinomas; most of the rest are cholangiocarcinomas (see Chapter 32).
- Tumors can be well-differentiated or poorly differentiated and focal or multifocal.
- Metastases occur through the tumor's ample vascular supply and may spread locally within the liver or into the portal vein or inferior vena cava (IVC).
- A subset of HCC, known as **fibrolamellar carcinoma**, affects younger individuals (20s to 40s) without prior liver disease and is histologically characterized by long bands of collagen alongside the neoplastic liver cells.

■ Clinical Manifestations

History

- Before HBV/HCV surveillance efforts, weight loss with right upper quadrant pain was the most common presenting symptom.

- Now, liver masses may be discovered incidentally in routine screenings.
- One should also consider the diagnosis of HCC in cirrhotic patients with sudden decompensation (e.g., sudden increase in abdominal girth and encephalopathy)

Diagnostic Evaluation

- Ultrasound (US) is widely used for screening patients with chronic HBV/HCV; it is less sensitive than computed tomography (CT) scan for smaller tumors (<1 cm).
- Because of the vascularity of HCC, three-phase CT scan classically shows enhancement on the arterial phase.
- α-Fetoprotein (AFP) is used in conjunction with US to screen carriers of HBV and HCV; it is about 50% sensitive and 87% specific for HCC (i.e., it can be normal in the setting of HCC; it is also elevated in the setting of germ cell tumors and sometimes necrotic liver diseases).
- An AFP level more than 400 with radiographic evidence of HCC is sufficient to make the diagnosis of HCC and to pursue therapy without tissue biopsy.

■ Staging

- Consensus has not been reached on the utility of current HCC staging models.

■ Treatment and Prognosis

- Surgery is the only therapeutic intervention that can achieve cure; the surgical options include resection and transplantation.
- Transplantation is possible in patients with a single tumor smaller than 5 cm or up to three tumors each smaller than 3 cm.
- Surgical resection is an option for rare patients with preserved liver function and small tumors (<10% of patients).
- Ablative therapies, in which an attempt is made to induce necrosis within the tumor, include radiofrequency ablation, percutaneous ethanol injection, hepatic artery embolization/chemoembolization, and laser therapy. These may be attempted when surgery is not a viable option; for small tumors (<3 cm), these therapies can approach the effectiveness of resection.
- Recurrence is common for resections and ablative therapies.
- Intra-arterial chemotherapy is generally reserved for inoperable patients with heavy disease burden and often consists of cisplatin, doxorubicin, and floxuridine.
- The overall median survival is 8 months.

Lung Cancer

■ Epidemiology

- Worldwide, lung cancer is the most commonly diagnosed neoplasm, but currently the incidence is higher in developed countries (e.g., North America and Europe).
- Lung cancer is more common in men than women; the highest rates are among African American men.
- Rates in women have risen rapidly since the 1970s; lung cancer is the most common cause of cancer-related death in American men and women.
- Adenocarcinoma has surpassed squamous cell carcinoma as the most common histologic subtype.
- For most lung neoplasms, incidence rates have reached a plateau in developed countries, likely as a result of smoking cessation patterns.

■ Risk Factors

- Tobacco use is responsible for about 90% of lung cancers; multiple epidemiologic, animal, and molecular studies have established this causal relationship.
- Smokers are at a 20-fold increased risk of developing lung cancer compared to nonsmokers; quitting significantly reduces but never completely erases the increased risk.
- Occupational exposures to carcinogens such as asbestos, arsenic, chromium, and nickel contribute to about 10% of lung cancers.
- There is a synergistic increase in lung cancer risk among persons exposed to both asbestos and tobacco.
- Radon, an inert gas emitted by soil into many homes and buildings, is thought to contribute to an additional 10% of lung cancer cases.
- Though controversial, passive smoking is thought to account for about 3000 cases of lung cancer yearly and is considered a known carcinogen by the United States Environmental Protection Agency.
- Increased consumption of fresh vegetables is associated with a lower risk of lung cancer, for reasons still unclear.

- β-Carotene supplementation was tested in cancer prevention trials and was found to be associated with a higher risk of lung cancer!

■ Pathology

- Small cell lung cancer, adenocarcinoma, squamous cell carcinoma, and large cell carcinoma together constitute about 90% of all lung neoplasms.
- Small cell carcinomas tend to originate centrally, grow rapidly, and metastasize early.
- Adenocarcinomas tend to be more peripheral lesions; they, too, metastasize early and are often accompanied by a malignant pleural effusion.
- Bronchoalveolar carcinomas are a subset of adenocarcinomas.
- Large cell carcinomas are typically large peripheral masses that may have cavitation.
- Smoking has been shown to contribute to all four major subtypes.
- Through the 1970s, squamous cell carcinoma was the most common histology; adenocarcinoma has now taken the lead as the most frequently diagnosed lung neoplasm.

■ Clinical Manifestations

History

- Classic presentation is of cough, with or without hemoptysis, dyspnea, or postobstructive pneumonia that does not resolve with antibiotics.
- Signs and symptoms suggesting more severe disease include chest pain (pleural or pericardial effusions), hoarseness, and Horner syndrome (superior sulcus tumors).
- Systemic manifestations are also common, including weight loss, fatigue, and the paraneoplastic syndromes.
- Patients, especially those with adenocarcinoma and small cell, may present with distant metastasis to the brain, adrenals, bones, or liver.
- Although there is no known genetic predisposition, some familial clusters have been documented.

Diagnostic Evaluation

- Workup of cough begins with a chest x-ray; large or unresolving pulmonary nodules should be biopsied.
- Sputum cytology, overall, is only 50% sensitive; for small cell lung cancer, it can suffice to make the diagnosis, although it is rarely useful in adenocarcinomas.
- Cytology of aspirated pleural fluid or of other metastatic foci is useful if positive.

- Central lesions (endobronchial or mediastinal) can be accessed and biopsied reliably through fiberoptic bronchoscopy.
- Peripheral lesions must often be biopsied either percutaneously (e.g., guided by computed tomography [CT]) or surgically via mediastinoscopy.

■ Paraneoplastic Syndromes

Syndrome of Inappropriate Antidiuretic Hormone

- Although a large percentage of small cell carcinomas secrete antidiuretic hormone (ADH), only about 15% of patients with the tumor have clinical syndrome of inappropriate secretion of ADH (SIADH), manifested by hyponatremia, euvolemia, and plasma hypoosmolality.
- Only about 30% of these patients are symptomatic (lethargy, confusion, seizures), likely because of the slow progression to hyponatremia.
- Effective chemotherapy usually leads to resolution within 2 weeks.
- Natriuretic proteins (e.g., atrial natriuretic peptide [ANP]) may also play a role in small cell carcinoma–related hyponatremia.

Humoral Hypercalcemia of Malignancy

- Parathyroid hormone–related peptide is secreted by about 20% of squamous cell carcinomas, accounting for elevated calcium levels in the absence of bony metastases.
- Symptoms include fatigue, altered mental status, gastrointestinal complaints, and polyuria.
- Humoral hypercalcemia of malignancy (HHM) is a poor prognostic sign, with median survival in affected individuals of only 1 month.
- Hydration and intravenously administered bisphosphonates (e.g., pamidronate) are the mainstay of therapy.

Ectopic Cushing Syndrome

- A small percentage (~2%) of patients with small cell carcinoma develop ectopic Cushing syndrome as a result of abnormal processing of proopiomelanocortin (POMC) with excess production of adrenocorticotropic hormone (ACTH) precursors.
- Clinically, these patients may have proximal muscle weakness, moon facies, hypokalemia, alkalosis, and hyperglycemia, but rarely the full-blown cushingoid phenotype.
- Ectopic Cushing syndrome is a poor prognostic indicator, with a median survival of only 4 months.
- Bronchial carcinoids can also lead to ectopic Cushing syndrome with increased ACTH and a more classic cushingoid presentation (hypertension, hyperglycemia, abnormal fat distribution, etc.).

Neurologic Manifestations

- Usually associated with small cell carcinomas, neurologic manifestation include paraneoplastic *Eaton-Lambert* syndrome, cerebellar degeneration, sensory neuropathy, and even encephalitis.

■ Staging

Traditionally, CT scanning of the chest, liver, and adrenals constitutes the staging workup. However, positron emission tomography (PET) scanning is increasingly being used to verify or exclude the presence of cancer in large mediastinal nodes.

The TNM staging method is used in the staging of lung cancers (Table 30-1); however, treatment and prognosis vary significantly between small cell and non–small cell carcinomas. If

---

■ TABLE 30-1 TNM Staging of Lung Cancer

Stage	Description
Stage IA	Tumor <3 cm surrounded by lung without invasion of bronchus
Stage IB	Tumor >3 cm without invasion of bronchus and >2 cm from carina
Stage IIA	Tumor <3 cm with ipsilateral hilar and/or peribronchial lymph node mets
Stage IIB	Tumor >3 cm with ipsilateral hilar and/or peribronchial nodes, or tumor of any size invading the chest wall, diaphragm, pleura, or pericardium or within 2 cm of the carina (T3)
Stage IIIA	Locally invasive tumor as above (T3) with ipsilateral hilar and/or peribronchial nodes, or tumor of any size (T1–T3) with ipsilateral mediastinal and/or subcarinal nodes
Stage IIIB	Any-size tumor with mets to the contralateral mediastinal, hilar, scalene, or supraclavicular nodes, or tumor invading heart, great vessels, trachea, esophagus, vertebral body, carina, or pleural fluid, with or without any nodes
Stage IV	Distant metastases

■ TABLE 30-2 Treatment and Approximate Survival Rates in Small Cell Lung Carcinoma

Stage	Description	Survival Rate
Stage I	Surgical resection and adjuvant chemotherapy	50% 5-yr survival
Stage II	Surgical resection and adjuvant chemotherapy	40% 5-yr survival
Stage IIIA	Neoadjuvant chemoradiation, surgical resection	20% 5-yr survival
Stage IIIB	Neoadjuvant chemotherapy ± radiation. Surgical resection if significant downstaging.	15% 5-yr survival
Stage IV	Combination chemotherapy	40% 1-yr survival

surgery is not an option, small cell carcinomas are defined simply as limited or extensive.

■ Treatment and Prognosis

- Small cell lung cancer (limited)—concurrent chemo/radiation. Consider prophylactic Cranial Irradiation in younger patients.
- Small cell lung cancer (extensive)—chemotherapy. Carboplatinum and Etoposide/CPT-11 is the standard of care.
- Non-small cell lung cancer—see Table 30-2.
- Neoadjuvant chemotherapy with radiation is usually a low carboplatinum dose (AUC2) and taxol or etoposide.
- Platinum doublets are the standard of care for metastatic disease. Example combinations are Carboplatinum/Taxol, Gemzar/carboplatinum, or Navelbine/Cisplatinum. Second line Texotere is approved for non-small cell lung cancer.
- Iressa and Terceva are approved for third and second line nonsmall cell lung cancer, respectively. These pills are epidermal growth factor receptor inhibitors. They have shown particular activity in women non-smokers and brochioalveolar histology. There is a possibility that patients with a mutation in the EGFR will prove to be the most responsive.

31 Ovarian Cancer

- Ovarian cancer is highly curable with early detection.
- Ovarian cancer is the most common cause of death among women who develop gynecologic malignancies, the second most common gynecologic malignancy, and the fifth most common cancer in women in the United States.
- Overall 5-year survival is about 50%.
- Epithelial cancers of the ovary account for more than 90%.

■ Epidemiology

- Disease of postmenopausal women.
- 50 to 75 years of age
- Whites: 15.4 per 100,000.
- 10.5 per 100,000 in African Americans.
- Highest rate in industrialized nations, although Japan is a notable exception. Highest rates in European-born Jews: 17.2 per 100,000.
- The etiology of ovarian cancer results from the accumulation of multiple discrete genetic events. A small proportion are from genetic syndromes; 10% result from BRCA-1, BRCA-2, and hereditary nonpolyposis colorectal cancer (HNPCC).

■ Risk Factors

- Average ovarian cancer risk in the United States is 1.5%.
- Higher fat consumption confers higher risk.
- Women with low parity are at an increased risk of ovarian cancer.
- Use of ovulation-inducing drugs for a prolonged period increases risk.
- Hormone replacement therapy has no clear association with increased risk.
- Marked protective effect with oral contraceptive pills (OCPs). OCPs can decrease the risk by 50% and the protective effect appears to last for years.

■ Hereditary Cancer Syndromes

- BRCA-1, BRCA-2, Lynch II/HNPCC, site-specific ovarian cancer syndrome.

- Clues to a patient with a cancer syndrome are multiple family members with the same malignancy or presentation at an early age.

BRCA-1
- Classified as a tumor suppressor gene.
- Mutations in this gene increase the risk of breast and ovarian cancer.
- Plays a role in repair of oxidative damage to DNA.
- BRCA-1 mutations are found in 1 in 800 in the general population and 1 in 100 in Jewish women of eastern European descent.
- Estimated lifetime risk of breast and ovarian in BRCA-1 carriers is 65% to 85% and 25% to 60%, respectively. This is compared to the average breast cancer risk in the U.S. population of 12.5% (1/8) and the ovarian cancer risk of 1.5%.
- A strong family history and a BRCA-1 mutation gives an even higher risk; increased to 90% and 65% for breast cancer and ovarian cancer, respectively.
- BRCA-1 may have a less aggressive course than sporadic cancers.
- BRCA-1 mutations are not a feature of sporadic ovarian cancer.

BRCA-2
- Tumor suppressor gene found less commonly than BRCA-1.
- Estimated lifetime breast cancer and ovarian cancer risk, respectively, of 65% to 85% and 15% to 25%, slightly lower ovarian cancer risk than BRCA-1.

Hereditary Nonpolyposis Colorectal Cancer
- Lynch syndrome.
- Increases the risk of ovarian, colon, breast, and endometrium cancer.

■ Clinical Manifestations
Early Stage Disease
- Insidious, producing essentially no symptoms.
- Abdominal pain 77%, gastrointestinal complaints 70%, constitutional symptoms 50%.
- Many times the symptoms are nonspecific abdominal discomfort.
- Cancers may grow very large (10 to 12 cm) before pushing on adjacent organs.
- May be incidentally detected as a pelvic mass. Imaging with ultrasound, computed tomography (CT), or magnetic resonance imaging (MRI) can detect the mass.
- About half of early ovarian cancers have elevated CA-125.

Advanced Stage Disease
- Abdominal bloating or swelling if ascites present.
- Large pelvic masses may produce bladder or rectal symptoms.
- Respiratory distress from pleural effusion, more common on the right side.
- Nodules may be palpated in the pelvic cul-de-sac on rectovaginal examination.
- Some patients with advanced cancer can have normal-size ovaries.

Diagnostic Evaluation
- No test, whether it be the CA-125 or the abdominal/transvaginal ultrasound, is *specific* enough to serve as a good screen.
- High false-positive rate with these tests.
- High-risk patients (hereditary syndrome carriers): periodic screening with CA-125 and sonography is recommended. Prophylactic oophorectomy after age 35 years if childbearing completed. Also, oophorectomy will lower the risk of breast cancer.
- Exploratory laparotomy is the usual way ovarian cancer is diagnosed.
- Preoperative evaluation is essential: history and physical, CA-125.
- If the patient is younger than 30 years, check B-hCG and AFP to rule out a germ cell tumor.
- Abdominal CT and MRI scans are useful in advanced stages.
- Preoperative evaluation of effusions is not necessary and can lead to seeding of tumor along tract of biopsy.

■ Pathology
- 90% are epithelial in origin, arising from the surface of the ovary.
- These cells give rise to various adenocarcinomas, including the following:
  1. Serous
  2. Mucinous: worse prognosis
  3. Endometrioid
  4. Clear cell types: worse prognosis
- Differentiation
  1. Grade 1: clear-cut glandular features, well-differentiated
  2. Grade 2: intermediate features
  3. Grade 3: solid sheets of tumor, poorly differentiated
- Grade of tumor correlates roughly with aggressiveness
- Stromal tumors: hormone producing, granulosa tumor, Sertoli-Leydig

---

■ BOX 31-1 Ovarian Cancer Staging

1. **Limited to ovaries**
   - 1A: limited to one ovary
   - 1B: limited to both ovaries
   - 1C: either 1A or 1B, but with tumor on the surface of one or both ovaries, capsule ruptured, ascites with malignant cells, positive peritoneal washings

2. **Growth involving one or both ovaries with pelvis extension.**
   - 2A: extension or mets to uterus or fallopian tubes
   - 2B: extension to other pelvis tissues
   - 2C: 2A or 2B, but with tumor on the surface of one or both ovaries, capsule(s) ruptured, ascites with malignant cells, positive peritoneal washings

3. **Involving peritoneal implants**
   - 3A: microscopic seeding of abdominal peritoneal surfaces
   - 3B: implants of abdominal peritoneal surfaces
   - 3C: abdominal implants > 2 cm

4. **Distant mets, pleural effusion with positive test result or liver mets**

Adapted from the American Joint Committee on Cancer Guidelines.

- Germ cell tumors: dysgerminoma, endodermal sinus tumor, malignant teratoma, embryonal carcinoma, and rare primary choriocarcinoma of the ovary

■ Staging

- Based on properly performed exploratory laparotomy by a highly trained gynecologic oncology surgeon.
- Box 31-1 outlines staging adapted from the American Joint Committee on Cancer guidelines.
- Surgery should include vertical incision, multiple cytologic washings, intact tumor removal, random peritoneal biopsies, including diaphragm washings, complete evaluation of all visceral and parietal surfaces, omentectomy, biopsy of aortic and pelvic lymph nodes, appendectomy, and hysterectomy with bilateral salpingo-oophorectomy. In some cases reproductive organ conservation can be accomplished.

■ Treatment

- Surgery affords best chance of a favorable outcome.
- For most patients, surgery is *not* curative because of dissemination throughout the abdominal cavity.
- Successful management requires additional treatment.
- Use of adjuvant chemotherapy is the standard of care for all patients with advanced stage disease and many patients with early stage disease and high-risk features.

- Adjuvant chemotherapy prolongs survival.
- The standard regimen is platinum and taxane (paclitaxel, docetaxel).
- Role of radiation remains unclear.

Treatment of Early Disease
- Comprehensive surgical staging for stage 1 and 2.
- Patients with 1A or 1B: Well-differentiated tumors have excellent 5-year survival rates of 90% to 98%. Adjuvant chemotherapy is usually not necessary.
- High-risk features include the following:
  1. Moderately to poorly differentiated tumors
  2. Stage 1C or 2
  3. Clear cell histology
- Survival rates are 60% to 80% for high-risk patients.
- Taxane and platinum chemotherapy should be considered a standard approach for patients with early stage disease and high-risk features.
- Optimum number of cycles is unclear, but three to four cycles is standard.
- Irradiation should be considered investigational.

Treatment of Advanced Disease
- Surgery: patients commonly found to have metastatic disease at the time of operation. Still important to document the surgical stage.
- Optimal cytoreduction: Primary function of surgery is debulking.
- Progression-free survival, median survival, and long-term survival are *all improved* in patients who have optimal cytoreduction.
- Even patients with residual tumors, those left with less disease, have a survival advantage.
- Survival advantage for platinum and taxane doublet compared to platinum-cyclophosphamide in advanced disease.

Treatment of Recurrent Disease
- Patients treated with the standard of platinum and taxane who relapse 6 months after completion of therapy often have additional responses of limited duration when re-treated with the same chemotherapy.
- Other chemotherapy options: topotecan and liposomal doxorubicin.

Pancreatic, Gallbladder, and Biliary Cancers

■ Epidemiology

- Pancreatic cancer is the fifth most common cause of cancer-related mortality in Western countries.
- Gallbladder and biliary tract cancers are relatively rare.
- The incidence for pancreatic, gallbladder, and biliary cancers peaks during the seventh decade.
- Pancreatic cancer is more common among men and blacks.
- Contrarily, gallbladder cancers are more common among women and Native Americans, Hispanics, and Alaskans; biliary tract cancers have no gender predilection.

■ Risk Factors

- Tobacco use is a risk factor for pancreatic cancer.
- Mutations activating the K-*ras* oncogene are found in most pancreatic cancers.
- Pancreatic cancer is associated with a few familial syndromes: hereditary pancreatitis, ataxia-telangiectasia, hereditary non-polyposis colorectal cancer (HNPCC), familial atypical mole-melanoma (FAMM), and Peutz-Jeghers.
- Cholelithiasis (especially with large stone), calcification of the gallbladder ("porcelain gall bladder"), and chronic typhoid carriage increase the risk of gallbladder cancer.
- Primary sclerosing cholangitis, ulcerative colitis, and chronic parasitic infections of the biliary tree predispose to bile duct cancers.

■ Pathology

- Most pancreatic tumors are ductal adenocarcinomas; rarer tumor types (~10%) include acinar, mucinous cystic, solid and papillary, neuroendocrine carcinomas, mesenchymal tumors, and lymphomas.
- Most gallbladder cancers are adenocarcinomas as well; accounting for about 15% are squamous cell and mixed tumor types.
- Biliary duct cancers are also most commonly adenocarcinomas; uncommon histologic types include carcinoid, adenosquamous, leiomyosarcoma, and mucoepidermoid carcinoma.

■ Clinical Manifestations

History

- Pain in the epigastric region or back and jaundice are the most common presenting features of pancreatic cancer; anorexia and weight loss are nonspecific symptoms.
  - A family history of breast, colon, or skin cancer should be elicited.
  - About 10% of patients with pancreatic cancer present with new-onset diabetes.
- Gallbladder cancer is usually asymptomatic until advanced stages, when patients may complain of right upper quadrant pain, nausea, weight loss, or jaundice.
- Most patients with bile duct cancers present with jaundice, although weight loss and pruritus are also common.

Diagnostic Evaluation

- Ultrasound is widely used as the first imaging study to evaluate jaundice.
- Computed tomography (CT) scan is the most accurate way to image pancreatic and gallbladder cancers, because it can visualize tumor extent and involvement of regional lymph nodes. CT scan with delayed imaging may pick up cholangiocarcinomas.
- Endoscopic retrograde cholangiopancreatography (ERCP) is the best way to explore and obtain tissue for diagnosis of biliary tract pathology.
- CA-19-9 is a useful marker for pancreatic cancer in terms of assessing the adequacy of resection and/or chemotherapy.

■ Staging

- The TNM staging systems are used in pancreatic and gallbladder cancers (Tables 32-1 and 32-2).
- Cholangiocarcinoma is staged based on invasion through the duct and into the periductal fibrous tissue and regional structures.

■ Treatment and Prognosis

Pancreatic Tumors

- Pancreatic tumors are considered unresectable if liver, peritoneal, or distal metastases is present; sometimes tumors involving the portal or mesenteric veins are still resectable.
- Unfortunately most of these tumors are unresectable.
- 5-year survival is about 33% for tumors less than 2 cm and locally invasive.
- 5-year survival is about 50% in the absence of regional nodal metastases.

TABLE 32-1 Overview of TNM Staging for Pancreatic Cancer

Stage	Description
Stage I	Tumor limited to the pancreas
Stage II	Tumor extends directly into the duodenum, bile duct, or peripancreatic tissue
Stage III	Tumor of either type listed above plus regional lymph node mets
Stage IV	Tumor extends into the stomach, spleen, colon, or adjacent large vessels with any nodal mets, or any tumor with distant metastases

TABLE 32-2 Overview of TNM Staging for Gallbladder Cancers

Stage	Description
Stage I	Tumor involves the mucosa
Stage II	Tumor extends into the muscularis
Stage III	Tumor extends through the muscularis
Stage IV	Tumor invades adjacent organs or liver mets found

- Adjuvant chemoradiation improves survival.
- Chemoradiation is the only option for unresectable; median survival is only about 8 months and drops to 4 to 6 months with distant metastases.

Gallbladder Tumors

- Gallbladder tumors are rarely resectable; in fact, stage I disease is usually found incidentally after cholecystectomy for other indications.
- These tumors are not very sensitive to radiation or chemotherapy.
- Overall 5-year survival is less than 5%.

Biliary Tumors

- Resectability decreases with more proximal lesions (i.e., nearer the intrahepatic ducts).
- Radiation may increase survival for unresectable disease (to median 24 months), but 5-year survival is still less than 10%.
- More published work is needed to evaluate the effectiveness of combination chemotherapy; the role of intrahepatic chemotherapy has not been defined for biliary tumors.

Prostate Cancer

■ Epidemiology

- Approximately 60% of men at autopsy have prostate cancer.
- The highest national incidence is found in the Scandinavian countries, the lowest in Asian countries.
- African American men are at the highest risk worldwide (10% lifetime risk).

■ Risk Factors

- The risk increases with age and African American ethnicity.
- The risk doubles in patients with affected first-degree relatives and increases exponentially with more than one affected first-degree relative.
- Low levels of selenium have been implicated by epidemiologic data in significantly increasing the risk of prostate cancer.
- No other purported risk factors are supported by consistent data.

■ Pathology

- Most prostate tumors are adenocarcinomas and histologically consist of well-differentiated glandular lesions.
- About 70% of these tumors occur in the peripheral zone of the prostate, often posteriorly, rendering them palpable via rectal examination.
- 20% of adenocarcinomas occur in the transitional zone and 10% occur in the central zone.
- Other rare tumor types include mucinous adenocarcinoma, transitional carcinoma, ductal adenocarcinoma, and small cell neuroendocrine tumors. Most of these have a poorer prognosis.
- Metastatic spread occurs through local invasion of lymphatics and blood vessels.

■ Clinical Manifestations

History

- Because most tumors occur peripheral to the urethra, patients usually remain asymptomatic until there is more advanced disease.

- Family history, focusing on first-degree relatives, is an important component of screening.
- Late-stage, larger tumors, or tumors arising near the urethra may present with symptoms of difficulty urinating, decreased urine stream, or nocturia.

Diagnostic Evaluation

- The **digital rectal examination** (DRE) can pick up nodules in asymptomatic patients.
- Transrectal ultrasound can be helpful in evaluating a nodule found on examination, especially for assessing local spread.
- The role of the **prostate-specific antigen** (PSA) for regular screening is controversial because of its high sensitivity and moderate specificity.
  - PSA is a protease produced by the prostatic epithelium and secreted into semen to liquefy seminal fluid on ejaculation; it is not normally secreted into the bloodstream.
  - PSA can be elevated in benign prostatic hyperplasia (BPH), prostatitis, and after prostatic manipulation (prostate massage, biopsy, possibly DRE).
  - The role of the PSA in following tumor response to therapy is important and a baseline PSA should be obtained in all patients with suspected prostate cancer who are amenable to treatment.
  - Otherwise healthy men older than 50 years should be offered the option of yearly PSA screening; high-risk patients should start at age 40 to 45 years.
  - Patients with PSA levels more than 4 should undergo biopsy, although the 4- to 10 range is considered a gray zone.
- **Transrectal biopsy** is the gold standard for making and confirming the diagnosis; the pathologist will generate a Gleason score based on tumor grade (1 through 10).
- Nomograms using the Gleason score and PSA help to determine treatment and likelihood of survival.

■ Staging

- The American Joint Committee on Cancer TNM staging system is used; in summary, it is as follows:
  - T1 and T2 tumors are confined to the prostate.
  - T3 and T4 tumors have local extension.

■ Treatment and Prognosis

Localized Disease (T1/T2)

- In patients who have a good life expectancy, radical prostatectomy is performed.

- The nerve-sparing procedure enables recovery of potency/erections in about 50% of men.
- Pelvic lymph node dissection is performed unless the patient is very low risk for disease outside the prostate (tiny primary, PSA < 10, Gleason < 7).
- These patients are usually observed without further adjuvant therapy unless there are positive lymph nodes or a rising PSA.
- **External beam radiation therapy** is an option for nonsurgical candidates and is usually combined with hormonal therapy (see "medical castration," in the following section).

Advanced Disease (T3/T4)

- T3 disease can be treated with surgery followed by adjuvant hormonal blockade, whereas metastatic disease is treated with castration alone to block the stimulating effect of testosterone on prostatic tissue.
- **Surgical orchiectomy** may be an option for persons not willing or able to take medications for the rest of their lives or who are intolerant of the meds.
- **Medical castration** is achieved through use of luteinizing hormone–releasing hormone (LHRH) agonists such as leuprolide or goserelin; these agents initially stimulate more testosterone release, but by overpowering the usual pulsatile release of LHRH, they feedback negatively to suppress further androgen synthesis.
- Flutamide, an antiandrogen, should be used at the start of LHRH agonist therapy to block this initial increase in testosterone.
- **Zoledronic acid** appears to be superior to other bisphosphonates for metastatic, hormone-refractory prostate cancer in terms of reducing bone pain, fractures, and osteoporosis.
- Docetaxel (Taxotere), based on two randomized studies, has shown a survival benefit.
- Vitamin D may have activity against prostate cancer; studies are ongoing.

34

Renal Cancers

■ Epidemiology

- Approximately 32,000 Americans are diagnosed with renal cancer each year.
- Incidence has been increasing every year for the past 20 years.
- The male/female ratio is 2:1.
- Incidence is higher in Scandinavians and North Americans; lower in Asians and Africans (although their incidence is also on the rise).

■ Risk Factors

- Smoking and obesity are both associated with increased risk.
- Increased risk with exposure to carcinogens such as lead phosphate, nitrosamines, and aflatoxin B_1.
- In patients on dialysis with acquired polycystic kidneys, up to 6% develop renal cancer.
- About 40% of patients with the autosomal dominant Von Hippel–Lindau syndrome (central nervous system [CNS] hemangioblastomas, pheochromocytomas, retinal angiomas) develop renal cell carcinomas (often bilateral and usually clear cell histology).

■ Pathology

- About 85% of all renal cancers are carcinomas (i.e., of epithelial cell origin); formerly known as hypernephromas, they are now thought to arise from the proximal tubules of the collecting ducts.
  - Of these, 75% are clear cell, 15% are papillary, and 5% are chromophobe.
  - **Medullary renal carcinoma,** a subset of the papillary carcinomas, is a rare (<1%) aggressive tumor that occurs predominantly in patients with sickle cell trait.
- **Oncocytomas** are also rare cell types (~5%) that are usually benign but occasionally have been found to metastasize.
- Transitional cell neoplasms of the renal pelvis/upper ureters account for 7% to 8%.
- Nephroblastomas account for 5% to 6% of all renal cancers.
- About 2% of renal cancers are sarcomas.

■ Clinical Manifestations

History
- Very few patients present with the classic triad of costovertebral angle pain, a palpable mass, and hematuria.
- Asymptomatic microscopic hematuria is the most likely finding in early disease.
- Unfortunately, most patients present late, with protean manifestations ranging from fever, malaise, and weight loss to paraneoplastic hematologic findings (see below).

Physical Examination
- Classically referred to as the "internist's cancer," the diagnosis is very difficult to make on physical examination until late in the disease process.

Diagnostic Evaluation
- Pursuing painless microscopic hematuria (found in ~65% of patients with renal carcinoma) with ultrasound and intravenous pyelogram (IVP) is essential in middle-aged patients.
  - Ultrasound is highly sensitive and specific in distinguishing benign from malignant renal cysts.
  - On IVP, look for distortion of the calyces or obvious mass lesions; this study is less sensitive for lesions of the posterior kidney or those that do not involve the collecting system.
- Patients may present with paraneoplastic syndromes such as hypercalcemia (from parathyroid hormone–like substance), hypertension, anemia (of chronic disease), polycythemia (from excess erythropoietin production), and polymyoneuropathy.
- Consider the diagnosis in a patient presenting with lung metastases of unknown origin, as more than 50% of renal carcinomas travel to the lung.

■ Staging and Prognosis

- Chest x-ray and computed tomography (CT) scanning, in addition to abdominal CT, are used to evaluate the size and extent of the tumor.
- Bone scan is indicated if the alkaline phosphatase level is elevated or the patient has bone pain.
- Head CT scanning is indicated only in symptomatic patients.
- A summary of the TNM staging system is shown in Table 34-1.

■ TABLE 34-1 Renal Cell Cancer Staging and Approximate Survival Rates		
Stage	Description	Survival Rate
Stage I	Tumors <2.5 cm confined to the kidney	95% 5-yr survival
Stage II	Tumors >2.5 cm confined to the kidney	88% 5-yr survival
Stage III	Either of the above with a single lymph node ≤2 cm, or tumor invades the renal vein or vena cava or adrenals or perinephric tissue but does not extend beyond Gerota's fascia	59% 5-yr survival
Stage IV	Lymph nodes >2 cm involved, or tumor extends beyond Gerota's fascia, or distant metastases present	20% 5-yr survival

■ Treatment

- Radical nephrectomy with regional lymphadenectomy is the cornerstone of therapy; surgical resection may be pursued with certain metastases.
- P-glycoprotein renders renal cell cancers resistant to most chemotherapeutic agents; radiation offers little or no benefit either.
- Some success has been noted with immunomodulation with interleukin-2.

Sarcomas

■ Epidemiology

- Sarcomas are rare malignancies that arise from tissue of mesenchymal origin, for example, bone, cartilage, fat, and connective tissue.
- Approximately 9000 new cases of soft tissue sarcomas are diagnosed each year in the United States, versus 2900 new cases of bone sarcomas.
- Men are affected more commonly than women at a rate of about 1.5:1.0.
- Osteosarcoma and Ewing sarcoma (bone) almost uniformly affect children and adolescents; the soft tissue sarcomas increase in incidence with age.
- There does not seem to be any racial preferences.

■ Risk Factors

- Increased incidence of soft tissue sarcomas in people with exposure to dioxins (emitted in waste combustion and found in herbicides, agent orange).
- Both bone and soft tissue sarcomas have been shown to arise in fields of previous irradiation, always at least 3 years after exposure.
- Both can also arise in patients treated with alkylating chemotherapeutic agents for other malignancies.
- Soft tissue sarcomas can arise in the setting of chronic lymphedema (e.g., filariasis); in women with chronic arm lymphedema after mastectomy, the development of such tumors is known as Stewart-Treves syndrome.
- Children with familial retinoblastoma have an increased risk of osteosarcoma.

■ Pathology

- For the most part, the exact cell type of origin of the non-bony sarcomas is not related to tumor behavior.
- Unless the tumor is well differentiated, it is often difficult to determine the cell of origin.
- 60% of soft tissue sarcomas arise in the extremity or superficial trunk, 15% in the retroperitoneum, 15% in the abdominal

viscera (intestines, uterus), and 10% in the head and neck region.

- **Osteosarcoma** is the most common primary bone tumor, followed by **chondrosarcoma** and then **Ewing sarcoma.**

■ Clinical Manifestations

History

- Most patients with soft tissue sarcomas present with a painless mass, whereas bone sarcomas tend to present with insidious pain and sometimes localized swelling.
- Although trauma to the involved region may initiate the diagnostic evaluation, trauma has not been shown to cause sarcomas.

Diagnostic Evaluation

- Beyond the physical examination, magnetic resonance imaging (MRI) is typically the imaging modality of choice for evaluating the origin and extent of sarcomas.
- Soft tissue masses greater than 5 cm persisting beyond 4 to 6 weeks should be evaluated by fine needle aspiration; retroperitoneal soft tissue masses are generally resected without preoperative biopsy.
- Bone sarcomas are diagnosed by biopsy, which should be performed by experienced surgeons to not interfere with future surgical plans.
- The first and most common site of metastases is the lung (the exception is visceral sarcomas in which the liver tends to be the first site of metastasis and thus should be imaged in the staging workup), so chest computed tomography (CT) scanning is usually performed as part of staging; however, negative chest x-ray findings in a patient with a soft tissue sarcoma smaller than 5 cm may suffice.
- For bone sarcomas, a bone scan is performed to rule out osseous metastases.

Staging and Prognosis

- Tumor size and grade constitute the basis for staging; soft tissue sarcoma staging also takes lymph node involvement into account.
- For osteosarcomas, poor prognostic factors include primary tumor of the axial skeleton, elevated alkaline phosphatase, and elevated lactate dehydrogenase.
- For soft tissue sarcomas, size more than 5 cm, high grade of tumor, and deep lesions are all poor prognostic factors.

■ Treatment

- Surgery is the mainstay of therapy, but adjuvant and neoadjuvant chemotherapy and radiation are increasingly being used in limb-sparing interventions.
- Chemotherapeutic regimens are usually doxorubicin based.
- New techniques aimed at delivering immunotherapy directly to the involved limb are under investigation and appear promising.

Skin Cancer

■ Epidemiology

- The skin is the most common site of cancer in the human body.
- The incidence of melanoma is on the rise; although the median age at diagnosis is 55 years, it affects many people during the second and third decades of life. It is the most common malignancy of American women between 25 and 29 years old.
- The incidence is slightly greater in men (1.2:1.0).
- Melanomas are most common in fair-skinned persons living closest to the equator; the incidence is highest in Australia and Israel.
- The non-melanomatous skin cancers are much more common but much less deadly.

■ Risk Factors

- Exposure to ultraviolet (UV) radiation (sunlight, especially ultraviolet B [UVB]) is associated with both melanomas and non-melanomatous skin cancers.
- Blistering sunburns early in life seem to predispose to melanoma, whereas non-melanomatous tumors tend to arise in areas of chronic sun exposure.
- There is a familial syndrome in which affected members have multiple atypical nevi (see below) and an increased risk of melanoma; the genetic underpinnings are not yet well described.
- **Xeroderma pigmentosa** is a rare disorder in which affected individuals lack the genetic repair mechanism to correct DNA damage caused by UV rays.

■ Pathology

- Malignant tumors may arise from any of the skin's cellular components:
  - Squamous cell carcinoma (SCC) and basal cell carcinoma both arise from epithelial elements.
  - Melanoma arises from melanocytes, which are the pigment-producing components of the skin.
  - The rare Merkel cell tumor arises from neural crest cells of the skin.

Squamous Cell Carcinomas

- Usually discovered early in sun-exposed areas and removed long before distant metastases arise.
- **Actinic keratoses** are lesions smaller than 1 cm in sun-exposed areas that are often sandpapery and can be red, tan, or brown; they are considered precursor lesions for SCC and can be burnt off with liquid nitrogen.

Basal Cell Carcinomas

- Basal cell carcinomas are also found in sun-exposed regions and are typically described as pearly papules, often with telangiectasias (dilated blood vessels).
- Microscopically, basal cell carcinomas often have a lymphocytic and fibroblastic infiltrate at their boundaries.

Melanomas

- Melanomas are most commonly found in women on the legs or back and in men on the back; other sites of origin include the eyes, anogenital mucosa, esophagus, and meninges.
- Atypical moles (atypical nevi or dysplastic nevi) are irregularly shaped, slightly raised brown moles larger than 6 mm that can develop into melanomas.
- Melanomas are usually pigmented, whereas non-melanomatous tumors are usually not.

■ Clinical Manifestations

History

- Patients should be instructed to note any changes in moles or freckles using the **ABCDE** mnemonic:
  - **A**symmetry
  - **B**order irregularity
  - **C**olor variegation
  - **D**iameter increase to more than 6 mm
  - **E**levation or ulceration of lesions
- A thorough family history of skin tumors should be documented.

Physical Examination

- Patients with atypical moles should have regular full-body skin examinations.
- Physical examination should include palpation of all lymphatic groups.
- Serial photography can be helpful in documenting lesions over time, especially when the patient has too many to biopsy.

Diagnostic Evaluation

- Any suspicious atypical moles or other lesions that exhibit the changes listed above must be biopsied.
- If the history and physical findings do not suggest disease beyond the lesion (i.e., asymptomatic, <1-mm deep/nonulcerative lesion, and no palpable lymph nodes), additional imaging and hematologic testing have very low sensitivity and specificity.
- Positron emission tomography scanning and lymph node ultrasound can be helpful if lymph node involvement is uncertain.
- Additional testing in the presence of nonlocalized disease may include chest x-ray, complete blood cell count, lactate dehydrogenase (LDH), and computed tomography scanning of the affected region.
- Brain magnetic resonance imaging should be pursued in the setting of headache or neurologic signs.

■ Staging and Prognosis

- The American Joint Committee on Cancer TNM system is used to stage melanoma (Table 36-1); the pathologic staging criteria are more involved than the clinical staging criteria but only really significantly influence survival data within the clinical stage III category.
- Among the various characteristics of a lesion, tumor thickness (depth) and ulceration have been shown to correlate most closely with tumor grade; thus, the T classification is based on these aspects alone.
- Without clinically apparent lymph node involvement, sentinel lymph node biopsy (SLNB) can be performed to determine the need for therapeutic lymphadenectomy (and if negative,

■ TABLE 36-1 TNM Staging and Approximate Survival Rates for Skin Cancer

Stage	Description	Survival Rate
Stage IA	Tumor ≤1 mm thick, no ulceration	95% 5-yr survival
Stage IB	Stage IA tumor with ulceration or up to 2 mm thick without ulceration	90% 5-yr survival
Stage IIA	Up to 2 mm with ulceration or 2 to 4 mm hick without ulceration	78% 5-yr survival
Stage IIB	2 to 4 mm thick with ulceration or >4 mm thick without ulceration	65% 5-yr survival
Stage IIC	>4 mm thick with ulceration	45% 5-yr survival
Stage III	Any T with any nodal metastases	27% to 65% 5-yr survival
Stage IV	Any T with any N and any distant metastases	6% to 19% 5-yr survival

sparing the patient the procedure's morbidity). In general, SLNB should be performed for lesions more than 1 mm deep, any ulcerative lesion, any lesion in a young patient, or high-grade lesions.

- The exact number of nodal metastases is part of pathologic, but not clinical, staging (one, two or three, and four or more).
- Note that serum **LDH** is associated with a higher M classification because it has been associated with more widespread disease, but this distinction does not change the clinical stage.
- Lung metastases have slightly better prognoses than the other visceral metastases, but this distinction does not change the clinical stage.
- Basal cell carcinomas almost never metastasize and SCCs do only rarely (~2%), usually after lymph node metastases are obvious.

■ Treatment

- Surgical excision is the mainstay of therapy for localized melanoma.
  - Excision margins for lesions less than 1 mm deep should be 1 cm.
  - Excision margins for lesions 1 to 4 mm deep should be 2 cm.
- For basal cell and squamous cancers, excision margins of 0.5 to 1.0 cm are adequate.
- Adjuvant therapy with interferon-α2b (IFN-α2b) has prolonged time to relapse.
- The use of adjuvant radiation therapy in melanoma is still controversial; however, in SCCs and basal cell carcinomas, success with radiation is nearly identical to that achieved surgically.
- Chemotherapy with the biologic agents interleukin-2 (IL-2) and IFN-α has had some success for metastatic disease.
- Chemotherapy with traditional agents can be used, but response rates are low.

Testicular Cancer

■ Epidemiology

- 95% of tumors in the testis are germ cell tumors, which can present in extragonadal primary sites.
- An estimated 7500 new cases are diagnosed annually.
- Testicular cancer is highly curable (>90%).
- Testicular cancer is the most common cancer in men aged 15 to 35 years, with a secondary peak after age 60 years.
- White men are affected more frequently, and it is rare in African Americans, with a 5:1 ratio.
- The highest incidence is in Scandinavia, Germany, and New Zealand; the United States is intermediate.

Genetic Marker

- Isochromosome of the short arm of chromosome 12p is detected nearly 95% of the time.

Extragonadal Tumor

- Approximately 5% of all germ cell tumors arise in the mediastinum, retroperitoneum, and pineal gland.
- Klinefelter syndrome (testicular atrophy, absence of spermatogenesis, gynecomastia), 47 XXY, is associated with primary mediastinal germ cell tumors.
- Hematologic malignancies (acute myelogenous leukemia subtype M7 megakaryocytic).
- Down syndrome (trisomy 21).

■ Risk Factors

- Prior testicular cancer; 3% will develop testicular cancer in contralateral testis.

Cryptorchidism

- No descent of the testis.
- Risk is 5 to 50 times higher .
- 10% to 15% of patients have history of cryptorchidism.
- 25% occur in contralateral testis that normally descended; pathophysiology is unclear.
- Early orchiopexy may decrease the likelihood of testicular cancer.

- Abdominal cryptorchid testis is more likely to develop cancer than inguinal.
- If testis is inguinal, hormonally functioning, and easy to examine, then watch.
- If not amendable to orchiopexy, then orchiectomy is recommended.

Fertility
- 40% have subnormal sperm counts before any treatment.

Not Risk Factors
- Prior trauma
- Elevated scrotal temperature: thermal underwear, jockey shorts, electric blankets
- Horseback riding or biking
- Diethylstilbestrol (DES) given to mothers of a male child
- Vasectomy
- Human immunodeficiency virus

■ Clinical Manifestations
- Painless testicular mass is the classic finding but usually seen in a minority.
- Most present with diffuse pain, ache, heaviness, swelling, or hardness.
- Hard to discriminate from epididymitis or orchitis.
- Acute pain, like testicular torsion, may represent intratumoral hemorrhage.
- 20% have associated hydrocele.
- Presentation in testis is the norm (90%).
- Extragonadal: 10% retroperitoneum > mediastinum > pineal gland.
- All patients with extragonadal site still need a testicular ultrasound.

Disseminated Disease
- Retroperitoneal disease usually presents with back pain or abdominal mass.
- Mediastinal disease presents with chest pain, cough, or shortness of breath.
- Can spread to supraclavicular lymph nodes.
- Hematogenous spread to lungs can present as cough, dyspnea, or hemoptysis.
- Can metastasize to brain.
- Bone pain is more common with seminoma.
- Metastatic disease to the liver presents as fullness and vague abdominal discomfort.

Diagnostic Evaluation
- First test to evaluate: testicular ultrasound; 95% of masses are malignant.
- Testicular biopsy is contraindicated; this may lead to aberrant lymphatic drainage to the inguinal and pelvic lymph nodes by local seeding.
- An inguinal surgical approach is preferred, a radical inguinal orchiectomy with ligation of the spermatic cord.
- Abdominal/pelvic computed tomography (CT) scan to evaluate lymph nodes.
- Chest radiograph should be performed or chest CT scan.
- Head and bone scans are unnecessary unless the patient is symptomatic.

Serum Markers
- Tumor markers are elevated in 80% of tumors.
- α-Fetoprotein (AFP), lactate dehydrogenase (LDH), human chorionic gonadotropin (hCG).
- AFP: single polypeptide chain, elevated in 50% of tumors
  - Half-life of 3 to 7 days; nonspecific; liver dysfunction, hepatitis, hepatocellular cancer, and other gastrointestinal (GI) tract cancers cause elevation.
  - Produced by liver, GI tract, fetal yolk sac.
  - Restricted to non-seminomatous histology.
- hCG: heterodimer, elevated in 60%
  - Half-life 24 to 36 hours.
  - Two subunits, α-subunit identical to leuteinizing hormone (LH), follicular-stimulating hormone, thyroid-stimulating hormone.
  - False-positive cross-reactivity with LH.
  - Produced by syncytiotrophoblasts.
  - False-positive test result with hypogonadism and recent marijuana use; false-positive test result occurs less frequently with newer assays.
  - Elevated in non-seminomatous and seminoma.
  - Can follow tumor marker levels after surgery and to monitor for disease progression.
- LDH: important prognostically independent of other markers

■ Histology

Carcinoma In Situ
- Precedes invasive testicular cancer.
- Frequently present in retroperitoneum.
- Median time to progression from carcinoma *in situ* (CIS) to cancer is 5 years.
- 5% of men with impaired fertility have CIS in cryptorchid testis.

- Testicular cancer is divided into two main categories: seminoma and non-seminomatous.

60% (Mixed)
- Embryonal: may have increase in hCG and/or AFP.
- Endodermal sinus (yolk sac): infants and young children; AFP level is usually increased.
- Teratoma.
- Syncytiotrophoblasts.
- Seminoma: When this tumor is mixed, it is treated as a non-seminomatous tumor.
- Choriocarcinoma: cytotrophoblasts and syncytiotrophoblasts; great propensity for hematogenous spread to lungs and skip retroperitoneum; hCG is usually high; hemorrhage into primary tumor is common.

30% (Pure)
- Seminoma usually appears in fourth decade of life.
- Strict definition of seminoma is to exclude the presence of any non-seminomatous type.
- 10% have focal syncytiotrophoblasts thought to be the source of hCG.
- **Note: No AFP elevation with seminoma.**
- Embryonal: Most undifferentiated with potential to become almost any cell type.
- Teratoma: composed of cell types from two or more germ layers: endoderm, mesoderm, ectoderm.
- Generally, teratoma is a benign tumor, but teratoma can grow locally and be lethal due to growing teratoma syndrome; compressive effects on surrounding organs.
- Mature teratoma: adult type differentiated cell type.
- Immature teratoma: partial somatic differentiation.
- Teratoma with malignant transformation: mature or immature teratoma that develops aggressive growth potential; must be surgically removed.

■ Pattern of Spread

- The pattern of spread is from the testis to the retroperitoneum, and then to the lungs or other visceral sites. Choriocarcinoma is known to skip the retroperitoneum and go directly to the lungs.

■ Staging (Table 37-1)

■ Treatment

Non-Seminoma Stage 1 (Confined to Testis and CT Negative)
- Radical inguinal orchiectomy first.

■ TABLE 37-1 Staging for Testicular Cancer	
Stage	**Cure Rate**
Stage 1: confined to testis, markers return to normal	100%
Stage 2A: <2 cm lymph nodes or markers elevated	98%
Stage 2B: 2 to 5 cm	
Stage 2C: >5 cm	
Stage 3: lung involvement or other	80%

- Choices then are as follows:
  1. Retroperitoneal lymph node dissection (RPLND)
  2. Surveillance

CONSIDERATIONS
- Risk of recurrence (usually retroperitoneal relapse) is 25%.
- 75% will not have nodal involvement.
- After RPLND, 10% to 15% will need additional treatment with chemotherapy.

SURVEILLANCE
- Careful meticulous follow-up.
- Patient compliance cannot be overemphasized.
- Chest x-ray, AFP, hCG, LDH, and physical examination monthly for 1 year, then every 2 months the following year, and every 3 to 4 months for the next several years.
- CT scan of abdomen/pelvis every 2 months during the first year, and every 4 months during the second year.

Non-Seminoma Stage 2 (Lymph Nodes Positive)
- Still need orchiectomy; because the testis is a sanctuary site and protected by the blood–testis barrier, chemotherapy will not penetrate.
- For masses/lymph nodes larger than 3 cm (high burden of disease), recommend chemotherapy.
- RPLND is recommended for the following:
  - Ipsilateral solitary lymph nodes 3 cm or smaller at or below the renal hilum, not associated with back pain, limited to the primary landing zone.
  - Surgical margins should not be compromised to preserve ejaculatory ability.
- After RPLND, chemotherapy recommended for the following:
  - High-burden disease: more than 6 lymph nodes, any node larger than 2 cm, or extranodal extension (high-burden disease).

Non-Seminoma Stage 2 (with High-Burden Disease) and Stage 3
- Orchiectomy using a radical inguinal approach
- Assess risk based on prognostic information given below

RISK ASSESSMENT

NON-SEMINOMA
- Good prognosis with all of the following:
  - AFP < 1000 ng/mL, hCG < 5000 U/L, and LDH < 1.5 times the upper limit of normal.
  - Non-mediastinal primary.
  - No non-pulmonary visceral metastasis; that is, the patient can have lung metastasis.
- Intermediate prognosis, all of the following:
  - AFP = 1000 to 10,000 ng/mL, hCG = 5000 to 50,000 U/L, or LDH = 1.5 to 10.0 times the normal
  - Non-mediastinal primary site
  - No non-pulmonary visceral metastasis
- Poor prognosis, any of the following:
  - AFP > 10,000 ng/mL, hCG > 50,000 U/L, or LDH > 10 times the normal
  - Mediastinal primary
  - Non-pulmonary visceral metastasis, for example, liver

SEMINOMA
- Good prognosis; no non-pulmonary visceral metastasis (bone, brain, liver)
- Intermediate (no such thing as poor risk in seminoma) prognosis: non-pulmonary visceral metastasis present

Treatment of Non-Seminoma Stage 2 (with High-Burden Disease) and Stage 3
- Good risk
  - Three cycles of bleomycin etoposide, cisplatin (BEP) or four cycles of etoposide and cisplatin (EP)
- Intermediate and poor risk
  - Four cycles of BEP
  - Controversy regarding optimal upfront chemotherapy for poor risk

Treatment of Seminomas
- Very sensitive to radiation

STAGE 1 DISEASE
- Radiation
- Side effects
  - Permanent infertility is rare.
  - Prolonged azoospermia more than 1 year may occur.

- Sperm banking recommended
- Simple para-aortic portal 2500 to 3000 cGy
- Elective prophylactic radiation to mediastinum contraindicated

Stage 2 Disease
- For infradiaphragmatic para-aortic and/or pelvic less than 5 cm, recommend radiation only.
- Larger lymph nodes require cisplatin-based chemotherapy.

Stage 3 Disease
- Chemotherapy is provided based on risk profile.

Chemotherapy Toxicities
- Cisplatin more efficacious than carboplatin; should not be substituted.
- Cisplatin induces delayed nausea.
- Nephrotoxicity is cumulative in all patients with cisplatin; effect is on proximal tubules.
- Long-term side effects of cisplatin include diastolic hypertension, increased low-density lipoprotein, decreased high-density lipoprotein, and increased weight gain.
- Auditory toxicity with cisplatin, including high-frequency hearing loss and tinnitus.
- Myelosuppression, neutropenic fever.
- Bleomycin pulmonary toxicity can be fatal! Review chest radiographs before cycles; Kerley B lines can be seen at lung bases on chest x-ray, rales heard at bases, decreased diffusing capacity for carbon monoxide, and difficulty with surgery and oxygen utilization.
- Cigarette smoking can cause late respiratory complications with bleomycin.
- Bleomycin can cause retroperitoneal changes as well.
- If bleomycin toxicity occurs, hold bleomycin and treat with steroids for 4 months.
- Raynaud syndrome occurs in less than 10% of those receiving bleomycin. Erectile dysfunction may occur as a result of microvascular insufficiency.
- Infertility is usually reversible. There is a 40% baseline infertility.
- Etoposide: Risk of leukemia with an 11q gene translocation; latency period for leukemia is 2 to 4 years.

38 Thyroid Cancer

■ Epidemiology

- Rare malignancies, constituting less than 1% of human cancers
- Median age at diagnosis 45 to 50 years.
- Approximate 3:1 female/male ratio
- Occult thyroid cancers found at autopsy in about 20% of adults

■ Risk Factors

- Irradiation to the neck in childhood increases the risk.
- Exposure to isotopes of iodine-131 as a result of the Chernobyl nuclear accident is thought to be responsible for the increased incidence of thyroid cancer in children who were younger than 10 years at the time of the accident.
- Three familial syndromes increase the risk for medullary thyroid cancer: familial medullary thyroid carcinoma and multiple endocrine neoplasia (MEN) types 2A and 2B.

■ Pathology

Papillary Carcinoma

- Papillary carcinoma is the most common histologic type of thyroid cancer; it originates from follicular cells and usually involves one lobe.
- May be multicentric within the lobe.
- Metastatic spread is through lymphatics.

Follicular Carcinoma

- Follicular carcinoma is the second most common type; it tends to be encapsulated.
- Metastatic spread is through blood vessels.
- **Hürthle cell** carcinoma is a variant with a poorer prognosis.

Medullary Carcinoma

- Medullary carcinoma originates from the parafollicular cells of the thyroid.
- Familial medullary carcinoma tends to be multifocal, and amyloid deposits are frequently found.

Anaplastic Carcinomas

- Anaplastic carcinoma is aggressive, with poorly differentiated tumors that often present as metastatic disease.

■ Clinical Manifestations

History

- Most patients with differentiated tumor types (follicular and papillary) present with painless thyroid nodules.
- Voice change may be a complaint when there is involvement of the recurrent laryngeal nerve or when the tumor is compressing the larynx.
- It is important to elicit any history of neck irradiation.
- Rapid size change is an important red flag (anaplastic carcinoma can present as a rapidly expanding neck mass)
- Most patients with thyroid carcinoma have normal thyroid hormone levels.

Diagnostic Evaluation

- Fine needle aspiration (FNA) is the diagnostic test of choice to determine the nature of a thyroid nodule.
- Ultrasound can help to identify whether a lesion is cystic or solid but cannot distinguish malignant from benign.
- Thyroid isotope scans determine the level to which the nodule takes up iodine; nodules that do not concentrate iodine are considered "cold" and have a higher rate of malignancy (only 10%) than "hot" nodules.
- Elevated calcitonin and carcinoembryonic antigen (CEA) levels are found in palpable medullary cancers.
- Germline mutations in the RET proto-oncogene are associated with most medullary cancers; children with the mutation should have thyroidectomy.

■ Staging and Prognosis

- The staging system for differentiated thyroid cancer is unique in that it takes age into consideration.
  - In general, low-risk patients are younger than 45 years with tumors smaller than 5 cm confined to the gland; they have about a 98% 20-year survival rate.
  - High-risk patients are those older than 45 years, with locally invasive or metastatic tumors or with large tumors (>5 cm; actually size cutoff debated); their 20-year survival rate is about 55%.
- Medullary cancers have an overall 10-year survival of about 50% (95% for tumors <1cm, <15% for metastatic tumors)
- Anaplastic carcinoma is, by definition, considered stage IV disease and the 5-year survival rates approach 0%.

■ Treatment

- Surgery is the mainstay of therapy for all types of thyroid cancer; total or near-total thyroidectomy is preferred, although lobectomy is sometimes done for very low risk patients.

- Therapeutic lymph node dissection is generally recommended for patients with papillary and medullary carcinomas; for follicular carcinoma, it is done only when lymph nodes are palpable or obviously enlarged on surgical exploration.

- Post-thyroidectomy radioablation with iodine-131 (radioactive) is recommended for patients with follicular and papillary carcinoma to kill any remaining thyroid tissue.

- Radiation therapy is useful for unresectable disease, particularly when residual disease does not take up iodine (as in medullary and anaplastic carcinomas).

- **Thyroglobulin** is a glycoprotein produced by follicular cells of the thyroid; it is very useful postoperatively in determining recurrence. Thyroid hormone replacement suppresses thyroglobulin levels, as do antithyroglobulin antibodies (check concomitantly); they are also lower when the thyroid-stimulating hormone level is suppressed. So, it is best to check thyroglobulin levels when the patient is off hormone replacement; if positive, consider repeating iodine-131 therapy.

39 Uterine Cancer

■ Epidemiology

- In the United States, the incidence of uterine cancer now exceeds that of cervical cancer at about 36,000 new cases per year.
- It afflicts African Americans less frequently than whites but is diagnosed at a later stage with lower 5-year survival rates in the former group.
- The median age at diagnosis is 61 years, with 80% of new cases in postmenopausal women.
- Approximately 5% of cases are detected in women younger than 40 years, usually in the setting of significant risk factors (e.g., polycystic ovarian syndrome [PCOS]).

■ Risk Factors

- Obesity (body mass index > 30) is a well-documented risk factor.
- Nulliparity, late menopause, and PCOS also increase risk, which are all thought to result in a relatively continuous exposure of the uterine lining to estrogen.
- Estrogen therapy in the form of tamoxifen or hormone replacement also increases the risk; the addition of progesterone, as in oral contraceptives, is thought to be protective against endometrial cancer, particularly in nulliparous women using them for more than 12 months.

■ Pathology

- There are five major histologic subtypes:
  1. Endometrioid adenocarcinoma constitutes the majority of uterine cancers.
  2. About 10% are adenosquamous carcinomas, which behave essentially like the endometrioid variant.
  3. Papillary adenocarcinomas are rare and clinically indistinguishable from the first two subtypes.
  4. About 10% are papillary serous carcinomas, which tend to present with invasion beyond the uterus and have a significantly poorer prognosis.
  5. About 5% are clear cell carcinomas, which tend to occur in older women and present at later stages.

■ **TABLE 39-1 International Federation of Gynecology and Obstetrics Staging System**

Stage	Description	Survival Rate
Stage I	Tumor confined to uterine body	>90% 5-yr survival
Stage II	Tumor invades the cervix	50% to 70% 5-yr survival
Stage III	Tumor invasion within the true pelvis (vagina, adnexa, peritoneal fluid)	20% to 40% 5-yr survival
Stage IV	Tumor metastases, including intra-abdominal or inguinal lymph nodes	<20% 5-yr survival

■ Clinical Manifestations

History

- Most patients present with postmenopausal or irregular menstrual bleeding.
- Assess for risk factors; regular physical examinations including bimanual and Pap smears are considered sufficient screening in the asymptomatic patient.

Diagnosis

- Outpatient endometrial biopsies have high sensitivity and specificity for making the diagnosis.
- Ultrasound is less accurate but is useful in demonstrating extrauterine spread of disease.

■ Staging and Prognosis

- Surgical staging has been found to be significantly more accurate than clinical/radiographic staging.
- Staging involves a total abdominal hysterectomy with bilateral salpingo-oophorectomy, peritoneal washings, and pelvic and para-aortic nodal sampling.
- The International Federation of Gynecology and Obstetrics (FIGO) staging system and estimated survival rates are summarized in Table 39-1.

■ Treatment

- Surgery is the mainstay of therapy.
- Stage I and II carcinomas are treated with adjuvant pelvic irradiation.
- Stage III is controversial; it may be treated with surgery and radiation, radiation alone, or combination chemotherapy depending on the extent of disease and tumor grade.
- Stage IV disease can be treated with chemotherapy; among the options are cisplatin plus doxorubicin.

Opportunities in Hematology and Oncology

The field of hematology and oncology ("heme-onc") offers myriad opportunities for the intellectually curious and patient care–oriented physician. In the private sector, the practicing specialist will deal largely with the most common malignancies—breast cancer, lung cancer, and colorectal cancer. The hematologic malignancies are much rarer and thus constitute a minority of the private oncologist's practice.

Private sector physicians in the cancer field must stay abreast of changes in the diagnosis, treatment, and management of malignancies. This involves attending national and local conferences, such as the American Society of Hematology and American Society of Clinical Oncology yearly meetings. Many larger private practices have also developed alliances with academic hospitals to enroll their patients in large clinical trials or to access highly specialized ancillary interventions (such as surgeries, radiotherapies, etc.).

Heme-onc is the perfect specialty for physicians who are committed to developing rapport and maintaining long-term relationships with their patients. The initial diagnostic and treatment pathway can be incredibly intense, with unexpected outcomes that range from disastrous to miraculous. The physician has an opportunity to guide, as well as to learn from, patients who are undergoing some of the greatest of life's challenges. Beyond identifying and administering the appropriate course of chemotherapy, the physician must anticipate and treat complications and develop a sense of when to modify a given protocol to better suit a given patient's needs and limitations. Addressing issues of death and dying can be quite rewarding for the physician who has won his or her patient's trust and esteem.

Another pathway in the field involves research. Because heme-onc is such an evolving field, there are ample opportunities in laboratory-based, translational, and clinical research. Medical school and residency are the appropriate times to try to get some exposure in these areas. In general, to seriously pursue a career in research, the physician should identify a specific area of interest early in the fellowship training. Graduating fellows might pursue research positions in biotechnology companies, in government-sponsored laboratories (such as the National Cancer Institute), or in the academic setting, where they must be able to obtain funding through large national funding sources (such as the National Institutes of Health). Depending on the university, the academic heme-oncologist can pursue a combination of research, teaching, and clinical practice.

It is possible to become board certified in hematology alone, although most private hematologists practice general internal medicine in addition to benign heme to stay busy. Academic specialists in larger centers can practice benign heme alone or some combination of benign and malignant heme, usually by incorporating research or running specialty centers (such as in sickle cell anemia). Benign hematologists receive various referrals for illnesses such as idiopathic thrombocytopenia purpura (most common), thalassemia, and sickle cell anemia. They are often asked to assist in the diagnostic pathway for leukocytosis, anemia, and thrombocytopenia.

The path to hematology and oncology involves completion of a 3-year residency training in internal medicine. Interested residents apply for a fellowship position during the second year of training. The fellowship is a 3-year commitment and most fellows subsequently take the national board examinations in both hematology and oncology. There are programs all over the country; larger university hospitals may have very separate hematology and oncology departments, and in smaller programs they tend to be fully integrated.

If you think you might be interested in heme-onc, be sure to visit a specialist practicing in the office because medical students and residents often see a very skewed version of the field by working only in the hospital setting. Malignancies are more often diagnosed and treated in the outpatient setting, often with excellent results. Unfortunately, patients who require hospitalization are often those with end-stage malignancies or severe complications caused by either chemotherapy or the cancer itself.

Good Luck!

Review Questions and Answers

QUESTIONS

1. A 52-year-old woman who had a hysterectomy 5 years ago is referred to you for persistent iron deficiency anemia that has not responded to iron replacement therapy. She reports normal appetite and normal daily bowel movements and except for mild exercise intolerance is asymptomatic. Her stool was negative for occult blood, and she has just had a colonoscopy, whose results were also negative. An endoscopy is scheduled for next week. Which of the following tests is most likely to suggest the diagnosis?

   A. Transferrin level
   B. Immunoglobulin A (IgA) antiendomysial antibody
   C. Vitamin B_{12} level
   D. Thyroid-stimulating hormone level
   E. Intrinsic factor antibody

2. A 41-year-old man with human immunodeficiency virus (HIV) comes to the emergency department (ED) complaining of hematemesis. His last CD4 count was 231 and he is not currently on highly active antiretroviral therapy (HAART). During his last clinic visit his hemoglobin level was 11.3, platelets 170,000, and pro-thrombin time (PT)/partial thromboplastin time (PTT) were normal. Currently, he appears agitated and is actively vomiting blood. He has an ecchymosis on his arm and his sclera appear icteric. He is also tachycardic. The rest of his physical examination in unremarkable. His platelet count is 13,000, his hemoglobin is 8.2, and his PT and PTT are very slightly elevated. The lactate dehydrogenase (LDH) level is 265. Which of the following pairs represents the next best diagnostic study and treatment plan?

   A. Hemoglobin electrophoresis—intravenous immunoglobulin (IVIg)
   B. Antiplatelet antibodies—plasmapheresis
   C. Peripheral smear—plasmapheresis
   D. D-Dimer/fibrinogen—intravenously (IV) administered heparin
   E. Reticulocyte count—upper endoscopy

3. A 15-year-old previously healthy white boy (English descent) is found to be anemic on routine laboratory tests taken for his sports clearance physical. He reports that his sister is also anemic. On physical

examination he has splenomegaly, but the examination otherwise is benign. He is discharged on a trial of iron and fails to return for his laboratory tests until 2 months later. The follow-up laboratory studies reveal a reticulocyte count of 5% with a persistent microcytic anemia. The Coombs test result is negative. Which of the following tests is likely to confirm the diagnosis?

A. Osmotic fragility test
B. Sucrose hemolysis test
C. Ham test
D. Hemoglobin electrophoresis
E. Heterophile monospot test

4. On your general medicine rotation, you are reviewing the laboratory results for a patient with lupus who presented with shortness of breath and was admitted to rule out a pericardial effusion. You notice an elevated PTT, normal PT, and slight anemia (hemoglobin = 11.9). Which of the following should be your next step?

A. Order a pure red blood cell (PRBC) transfusion
B. Initiate heparin therapy
C. Order a reticulocyte count
D. Order a transfusion of fresh frozen plasma (FFP)
E. Order a 50:50 mixing study for PTT

5. A 54-year-old woman presents with chronic postprandial epigastric pain. *Helicobacter pylori* immunoglobulin G (IgG) antibody is positive. Endoscopy reveals diffuse gastritis with a thickened area of gastric mucosa that is biopsied. Results reveal a mucosa-associated lymphoid tissue lymphoma ("MALToma"). Which of the following pairs represent the most appropriate initial therapy and clinical outcome?

A. Treat *H. pylori* infection—prompt permanent eradication of malignancy
B. Perform gastrectomy—distant metastases inevitable
C. Treat *H. pylori* infection—eradication of malignancy over 2-year period, chemotherapy effective at preventing recurrence
D. Initiate chemotherapy—persistent *H. pylori* antibodies suggest metastatic disease
E. Initiate proton pump inhibitor—eradication of MALToma with chronic acid suppression

6. A 54-year-old man presents with fatigue and early satiety. On physical examination he is pale with splenomegaly. Laboratory study results reveal a white blood cell (WBC) count of 89,000, with neutrophilia but without blasts. Hemoglobin level is 9.9. Which of the following pairs represent the goal of initial and long-term therapy in this patient?

A. Reduce the WBC count—eradicate Bcr-Abl translocation
B. Raise the hemoglobin level—reduce the WBC count
C. Reduce the WBC count—raise the hemoglobin level

   D. Watchful waiting—bone marrow transplant
   E. Watchful waiting—reduce the WBC count when symptomatic

7. In which of the following groups of cancer has tobacco been clearly implicated as a risk factor?

   A. Pancreatic, gastric, hepatic, lung, and bladder
   B. Head and neck, lung, pancreatic, renal, and bladder
   C. Esophageal, oropharyngeal, nasopharyngeal, biliary, and lung
   D. Sarcoma, lung, breast, oropharyngeal, and gastric
   E. Biliary, breast, throat, bladder, and gastric

8. A 41-year-old woman with a history of melanoma resected about 9 months ago presents with headache, slurred speech, and left-sided weakness. Computed tomography (CT) scan of the head reveals multiple lesions, the largest in the right frontotemporal region with significant surrounding edema that is causing midline shift. What is the most appropriate initial therapy?

   A. Magnetic resonance angiography (MRA) of the brain to rule out vasculitis
   B. Emergent chemotherapy
   C. Admit the patient for intracranial biopsy
   D. Administer intravenous dexamethasone immediately
   E. Emergent IV administered mannitol

9. A 71-year-old woman with no history of bleeding presents complaining of progressive fatigue, easy bruisability, and gum bleeding. On physical examination, she is pale, with scattered ecchymoses and oral petechiae. Laboratory studies reveal a platelet count of 100,000, low hemoglobin level (8.1 mg/dL), and elevated blood urea nitrogen (BUN) and creatinine (45/2.8). The total protein is 8.2, albumin 2.0, total bilirubin 0.9, and normal liver enzymes. Which of the following is the most likely cause of this patient's gum bleeding?

   A. Acquired defect in platelet function
   B. Thrombocytopenia
   C. Thrombotic thrombocytopenic purpura (TTP)
   D. Acquired hemophilia
   E. von Willebrand disease

10. A 22-year-old man with a 2-month history of cough is referred to you because his chest x-ray (CXR) reveals a large mediastinal mass. CT scans of chest, abdomen, and pelvis reveal only a few enlarged retroperitoneal lymph nodes. Which of the following complete your initial workup as you wait for the biopsy results?

   A. Thorough skin examination, carcinoembryonic antigen (CEA), thyroglobulin, LDH
   B. Thorough skin examination, LDH, prostate-specific antigen (PSA)
   C. Thorough testicular examination, LDH, thyroglobulin, and fluorescence *in situ* hybridization (FISH) for Bcr-Abl

    D. Thorough testicular examination, LDH, α-fetoprotein (AFP), and human chorionic gonadotropin (hCG)

    E. Thorough thyroid examination, TSH, thyroglobulin

11. A 56-year-old female smoker presents to you with a 3-month history of severe frontal headaches. She has no focal neurologic findings, and other than injected conjunctiva, her physical examination is unremarkable. Her laboratory findings are normal except for a hemoglobin level of 19 and 2+ RBCs on urine dipstick. What malignancy are you concerned about?

    A. Lung cancer

    B. Renal cell carcinoma

    C. Bladder cancer

    D. Intracranial neoplasm

    E. Lymphoma

12. You are evaluating a 69-year-old man in your general medicine office. He reports feeling well except for a cough that started about 6 months ago. He quit smoking around the same time, denies headache, and states that the cough has not interfered with physical activities such as mowing the lawn, climbing stairs, etc. On physical examination, he is a muscular man who appears in good health except for occasional end-expiratory wheezes noted on lung examination. His laboratory examination reveals slight anemia (hemoglobin = 12.2) and a sodium level of 133. Which of the following pairs represents the most important next diagnostic study and presumed diagnosis?

    A. Head CT—metastatic cancer

    B. Serum osmoles—syndrome of inappropriate secretion of antidiuretic hormone (SIADH)

    C. CXR—small cell lung cancer

    D. CXR—pneumonia

    E. Chest CT—squamous cell lung cancer

13. A 42-year-old female smoker presents with a small breast mass that, on fine needle aspiration (FNA), reveals lobular carcinoma *in situ* (LCIS). Which of the following do you tell her about this diagnosis?

    A. This is a benign lesion that is of little concern.

    B. She has an increased risk for uterine cancer.

    C. She has an increased risk for breast cancer in either breast.

    D. If she quits smoking, the lesion will most likely regress.

    E. She must have a bilateral therapeutic mastectomy.

14. A 60-year-old woman presents with mammogram findings that reveal microcalcifications that, on biopsy, were consistent with ductal carcinoma *in situ* (DCIS). What do you recommend?

    A. Lumpectomy with radiation and tamoxifen therapy

    B. Modified radical mastectomy on the affected side

    C. Delay recommendation until an axillary lymph node dissection is performed

    D. Start therapy with tamoxifen

    E. Watchful waiting with repeated mammogram in 3 months

15. Which of the following screening tests is most likely to reduce over-all mortality from cancer?

    A. Digital rectal examination for colorectal cancer

    B. PSA for prostate cancer

    C. CA-19-9 for pancreatic cancer

    D. Yearly CXRs in smokers

    E. Pap smear for cervical cancer

16. Which of the following is not a risk factor for hepatocellular carcinoma?

    A. Chronic infection with hepatitis B and C viruses

    B. Aflatoxin B

    C. Hemochromatosis

    D. Alcoholism

    E. Chronic infection with *Clonorchis sinensis*

17. An 18-year-old boy presents with a dull ache in his right testicle. An ultrasound is positive for a testicular mass. Which of the following is the correct pairing of the testicular germ cell tumor type and its serum marker?

    A. Pure seminoma—elevated AFP, elevated β-hCG

    B. Pure seminoma—normal to slightly elevated β-hCG, normal AFP

    C. Nonseminoma—normal AFP, elevated β-hCG

    D. Nonseminoma—low AFP, low β-hCG

    E. Nonseminoma—normal AFP, elevated LDH

18. An 81-year-old man with a 6-month history of worsening back pain is evaluated by his primary medical doctor and is found to have a PSA of 156. Which of the following pairs best represents the type of bony lesions and the appropriate study to visualize them in this patient?

    A. Osteoblastic—nuclear bone scan

    B. Osteoclastic—skeletal series

    C. Osteoblastic—bone densiometry

    D. Osteoclastic—nuclear bone scan

    E. Osteoblastic—skeletal series

19. A 72-year-old woman who had right breast cancer diagnosed 25 years ago and was treated with radical mastectomy with axillary lymph node dissection presents to you complaining of a "bump" that she noticed about 2 months ago when she banged her arm while cleaning. She states that her arm has been chronically swollen ever since the breast surgery, and although the lesion is not very painful, it seems to be growing. Which of the following complications are you concerned about?

    A. Deep venous thrombosis (DVT)

    B. Phlebitis

    C. Recurrent breast cancer

D. Sarcoma

E. Abscess

20. A 32-year-old woman presents with a dark-red skin lesion on her left arm, which has grown and become asymmetric over the last 2 months. Biopsy by an outside dermatologist revealed a melanoma of 3 mm depth. The surgical intern is uncertain how to proceed and asks for your advice on the surgical margins. What do you tell her?

A. A melanoma of this depth requires 3-mm margins.

B. A melanoma of this depth requires 1-cm margins.

C. A melanoma of this depth requires 2-cm margins.

D. A melanoma of this depth requires 3-cm margins.

E. A melanoma of this depth requires 5-cm margins.

21. A 17-year-old girl is admitted to your service complaining of bright red blood per rectum. She is found to have a hemoglobin level of 8.9. A colonoscopy is performed, revealing multiple ulcerations extending from the rectum to the splenic flexure. Medications for ulcerative colitis are initiated with adequate control of her bloody diarrhea. She read up on the topic on the Internet and wants to know how you will go about colorectal cancer surveillance in her. What do you tell her?

A. She should have a prophylactic colectomy as soon as possible.

B. She should have yearly colonoscopies.

C. She should begin to have yearly colonoscopies in about 8 to 10 years.

D. No surveillance is necessary.

E. She should have surveillance colonoscopies every 3 years.

22. You are evaluating a 67-year-old man in your general medicine clinic for fatigue. A complete blood cell (CBC) count reveals a WBC count of 16,000 with neutrophilia. Which of the following laboratory results would lead you to evaluate him further for chronic myelogenous leukemia (CML)?

A. An elevated erythrocyte sedimentation rate (ESR)

B. An elevated leukocyte alkaline phosphatase

C. An elevated creatinine

D. A low reticulocyte count

E. A low leukocyte alkaline phosphatase

23. An 18-year-old woman complaining of drenching night sweats and a 16-pound weight loss is admitted to your service. On physical examination you detect several enlarged lymph nodes in the axillary, cervical, and supraclavicular regions. A CT scan of the chest, abdomen, and pelvis reveal additional mediastinal lymphadenopathy. An excisional biopsy of a lymph node reveals numerous Reed-Sternberg cells. The bone marrow biopsy is negative for involvement. What do you inform the patient?

A. She has stage IIB non-Hodgkin lymphoma (NHL).

B. She has stage IIA NHL.

C. She has mononucleosis.

D. She has stage IIB Hodgkin lymphoma.

E. She has stage III Hodgkin lymphoma.

24. A 58-year-old man from the Philippines presents with symptoms suggestive of cirrhosis. On physical examination, his skin appears much darker than that of his family members and a liver edge is palpable 4 cm below the costal margin. He has some swelling and tenderness of the bilateral metacarpophalangeal (MCP) joints of his hands. Laboratory evaluation reveals an elevated glucose, low albumin, slightly elevated PT and activated PTT (aPTT), and a hemoglobin of 11g/dL. The patient admits to a history of melena, so you order iron studies to rule out iron deficiency and are surprised to find that the ferritin level is 677 µg/mL and saturation is 92%. He has not received a blood transfusion. What do you do next?

A. Request a liver biopsy to rule out hemochromatosis

B. Discuss privately his history of alcohol use

C. Perform phlebotomy

D. Request an HFE gene mutation study to rule out hemochromatosis

E. Nothing

25. A 49-year-old woman with a history of rectal prolapse is awaiting surgery. You are called by the blood bank because the patient's blood was found to have anti-E and anti-C antibodies. What do you recommend to the surgeons regarding the use of blood transfusion during surgery?

A. Antibodies against these minor antigens should not cause a problem.

B. Use only E-antigen– and C-antigen–negative blood.

C. A hemolytic reaction is likely if this patient is Rh positive.

D. The patient likely has a chronic hemolytic anemia and should be transfused before surgery.

E. Avoid blood transfusion at all costs.

ANSWER KEY

1. B	10. D	19. D
2. C	11. B	20. C
3. A	12. C	21. C
4. E	13. C	22. E
5. C	14. A	23. D
6. A	15. E	24. A
7. B	16. E	25. B
8. D	17. B	
9. A	18. A	

ANSWERS

1. **B.** Up to 5% of patients with iron deficiency anemia have celiac sprue, which can be diagnosed by small bowel biopsy. **IgA antiendomysial antibodies are highly sensitive and specific, making them a good screening test.**

2. **C. The peripheral smear is invaluable in making the diagnosis of TTP. Schistocytes on the smear represent mechanical destruction of red cells.** The patient's scleral icterus and abrupt drop in hemoglobin and platelet count are highly suggestive of the diagnosis, especially in the setting of HIV. The LDH is elevated as a result of hemolysis. Treatment with plasmapheresis/plasma exchange transfusion should be initiated as soon as possible in patients with TTP.

3. **A. This patient most likely has hereditary spherocytosis. The peripheral blood examination would reveal small, round red blood cells.** Clues include the patient's splenomegaly and positive family history. β-Thalassemia is another possibility and would be diagnosed by hemoglobin electrophoresis; however, this patient is white and the thalassemias are more likely to occur in people of African, Mediterranean, and Asian descent.

4. **E. This patient with lupus has an elevated PTT. The initial workup for an elevated PTT, after repeating the test to confirm the abnormality, is to order a 50:50 mixing study in which normal serum is combined with the patient's and retested for PTT.** If the value corrects, the patient has a deficiency in one of the clotting factors of the intrinsic pathway which can cause bleeding. If it does not correct, the patient has an inhibitor such as lupus anticoagulant or anti-cardiolipin antibodies, both of which are more common in patients with lupus. If so, this patient's shortness of breath may be due to a pulmonary embolus rather than a pericardial effusion!

5. **C.** Eradication of *H. pylori* infection has been associated with regression of gastric MALTomas. However, chemotherapy is usually still used to suppress recurrence. Similarly, eradication of hepatitis C virus has been associated with regression of splenic lymphoma.

6. **A.** The immediate goal in this patient with CML is to reduce the WBC count to prevent complications such as hyperviscosity syndrome. This can be achieved with hydroxyurea; allopurinol and hydration should be given to reduce the risk of gout from rapid cell death. The only "cure" for CML is still considered bone marrow transplant. However, the use of Gleevec (tyrosine kinase inhibitor STI 571) has resulted in eradication of the Bcr-Abl translocation defect. Long-term efficacy is still under study.

7. **B.** Of the above, only sarcomas, biliary, and hepatic cancers have not been related to tobacco smoking.

8. **D.** The differential diagnosis for multifocal intracranial lesions is vasculitis, infection, and metastases. Given the history of melanoma, the latter is most likely. In the setting of a mass effect, impending herniation, or significant edema with focal neurologic findings, the first therapeutic intervention should be IV administered dexamethasone. The radiation oncologists and neurosurgeons should be notified as soon as possible (ASAP) in cases such as this one.

9. **A.** This patient, who most likely has multiple myeloma, has at least two problems that may be inhibiting her platelets. Uremia can interfere with platelet adhesion and aggregation. The elevated globulin fraction (8.2 − 2.0 = 6.2) can also inhibit platelet aggregation by coating the platelets or by resulting in autoantibodies against platelet antigens or factors necessary for clotting.

10. **D.** Based on his age, the most likely cancer diagnoses would be lymphoma, testicular cancer, and melanoma. The lymphadenopathy and mediastinal mass could occur in either lymphoma or testicular cancer. Given the patient's age and sex, and because testicular cancer metastasizes to retroperitoneal nodes, it is essential to rule this out.

11. **B.** The presence of erythrocytosis may be secondary to smoking-induced lung disease or chronic sleep apnea. However, in a smoker with microscopic hematuria, erythrocytosis can represent inappropriate erythropoietin secretion by a renal cell carcinoma. Other tumors that can secrete erythropoietin include hepatocellular carcinomas and cerebellar hemangiomas. But, this patient's presentation is not consistent with either of these.

12. **C.** The most important next step is to rule out lung cancer as the etiology of SIADH in this older male smoker with a cough. Small cell lung cancer is the histology associated with SIADH. The hyponatremia is mild and asymptomatic and will usually resolve with treatment of the cancer.

13. **C. LCIS is considered a marker for malignancy because approximately 30% of affected patients will develop breast cancer in the same or contralateral breast.** Tamoxifen has been effective chemoprophylaxis in these patients; because lesions are often multifocal, some women may choose prophylactic mastectomy.

14. **A.** DCIS is also strongly associated with recurrence of breast cancer, even after surgical excision. However, prophylactic mastectomy is probably overkill, unless it is requested by the patient. **Treatment with radiation and tamoxifen therapy after lumpectomy appears to reduce the recurrence rates appreciably, making lumpectomy a viable option.**

15. **E. Of the choices, only the Pap smear seems to actually reduce cancer mortality.** In some developing countries where access to routine health care is poor and Pap smears are not commonly performed, cervical cancer is still a leading cause of death for women.

16. **E.** All of the above are risk factors for liver cancer except infection with the fluke Clonorchis. That is a risk factor for cholangiocarcinoma.

17. **B. Whenever the AFP is elevated in the setting of testicular cancer, the tumor is considered a nonseminomatous germ cell tumor.**

18. **A. Metastatic prostate cancer is associated with osteoblastic lesions, which can be well visualized on bone scan because they take up the compound.** Osteoclastic lesions, as seen in multiple myeloma, do not typically show up on bone scans.

19. **D. Chronic lymphedema, as in women who have had axillary lymph node dissections for breast cancer, can predispose to sarcoma in the affected arm.** DVT would not present as an enlarging, painless mass. Phlebitis would occur soon after intravenous placement and would present as a tender region overlying the vein. Recurrent breast cancer would be very unusual in the arm. An abscess would be unlikely to have such an indolent course.

20. **C. For melanoma, surgical margins should be 1 cm for lesions less than 1 mm depth, and 2 cm for lesions 1 to 4 mm in depth.**

21. **C. Patients with ulcerative colitis have an increased risk of colorectal cancer. Surveillance colonoscopies should begin about 8 years after pancolitis is diagnosed and repeated every 1 to 2 years thereafter. Any sign of dysplasia should prompt an elective colectomy.**

22. **E. In patients with elevated WBC counts, the leukocyte alkaline phosphatase can be used to help distinguish between infection and CML, as it is elevated in the former and low in the latter.**

23. **D. Reed-Sternberg cells are the classic finding in Hodgkin lymphoma. This patient has several lymph node groups all on one side of the diaphragm along with "B" symptoms of sweats and weight loss, which make her disease stage IIB.**

24. **A.** Hemochromatosis is suggested by the physical examination findings (bronze skin, enlarged liver, small joint arthritis) and by the laboratory results (diabetes, early cirrhosis, elevated ferritin, and elevated iron saturation). **The definitive diagnosis is made by performing a liver biopsy.**

25. **B.** As long as the blood bank knows that the patient may need a transfusion, donor blood can be screened for antigens to which the patient has antibodies and appropriate antigen-negative blood can be given if necessary.

C Hematologic/Oncologic Medications and Toxicities

Chemotherapy drugs can be divided into cell cycle specific or not.

Cell Cycle

- G_1: Postmitotic period, a phase when enzymes necessary for DNA production, proteins, and RNA are produced.
- S: DNA synthesis, all DNA synthesis takes place.
- G_2: Premitotic period, more protein and RNA synthesis occurs.
- M: mitosis, physical division takes place. Two daughter cells are formed and again each one enters to G_1.
- G_0: Cells relatively inactive.

Cell Cycle Active but Not Phase Specific

- Alkylating agents: cross-linking of DNA strands.
- General toxicities: Gonadal, teratogenic, myelosuppression, secondary malignancy.
- See Table C-1 for examples.

Cell Cycle Active and Phase Specific

■ S-Phase Specific

- Antimetabolites: structural analogues of normal molecules; interfere with DNA synthesis.
- See Table C-2 for examples.

■ G_2-Phase Specific

- Antitumor antibiotics: interfere with DNA synthesis.
- See Table C-3 for examples.

■ M-Phase Specific

- Mitotic spindle agents: inhibit the mitotic spindle.
- See Table C-4 for examples:

■ TABLE C-1

Drug	Main Side Effects
Busulfan	Myelosuppression, pulmonary fibrosis
Chlorambucil	Myelosuppression
Cyclophosphamide	Myelosuppression, hemorrhagic cystitis
Ifosfamide	Myelosuppression, hemorrhagic cystitis
Melphalan	Myelosuppression, stem cell damage
Nitrogen mustard	Myelosuppression
Nitrosoureas	Myelosuppression, pulmonary fibrosis
Streptozocin	Nephrotoxicity
Thiotepa	Myelosuppression
Cisplatin	Myelosuppression, renal insufficiency, neurotoxicity, ototoxicity
Carboplatin	Myelosuppression, renal insufficiency
Oxaliplatin	Cold neuropathies, neutropenia
Dacarbazine	Myelosuppression
Procarbazine	Myelosuppression
Temozolomide	Myelosuppression

■ TABLE C-2

Drug	Main Side Effects
Azacitidine	Myelosuppression, neurotoxicity
Cladribine	Myelosuppression
Cytarabine	Myelosuppression, cerebellar toxicity
Fludarabine	Myelosuppression, immunosuppression
Fluorouracil	Myelosuppression, diarrhea
Leucovorin	None
Capecitabine	Diarrhea, hand-foot syndrome
Gemcitabine	Myelosuppression, pulmonary effects
Hydroxyurea	Myelosuppression, painful ulcers
Mercaptopurine	Myelosuppression
Methotrexate	Myelosuppression, renal dysfunction, liver abnormalities
Pentostatin	Myelosuppression, immunosuppression

■ TABLE C-3

Drug	Main Side Effects
Actinomycin D	Myelosuppression
Bleomycin	Myelosuppression, pulmonary disease, dermatologic, Raynaud disease
Doxorubicin	Myelosuppression, cardiomyopathy
Epirubicin	Myelosuppression, cardiomyopathy
Idarubicin	Myelosuppression, cardiomyopathy
Mitomycin	Myelosuppression
Mitoxantrone	Myelosuppression, cardiomyopathy

■ TABLE C-4

Drug	Main Side Effects
Paclitaxel	Myelosuppression, peripheral neuropathy, hypersensitivity
Docetaxel	Myelosuppression, hypersensitivity
Vinblastine	Myelosuppression, neurotoxicity
Vincristine	Myelosuppression, neurotoxicity
Vinorelbine	Myelosuppression

■ TABLE C-5

Drug	Main Side Effects
Irinotecan	Diarrhea, myelosuppression
Topotecan	Myelosuppression
Etoposide	Myelosuppression

■ TABLE C-6

Drug	Main Side Effects
Interferon	Renal failure
Interleukin-2	Severe capillary leak syndrome, renal failure

Topoisomerase Inhibitors (Table C-5)

Biologic Agents (Table C-6)

Monoclonal Antibodies

- Rituxan: monoclonal antibody directed against CD20 on lymphocytes
  - Anti-HER-2/neu murine monoclonal antibody with human Fc region and heavy chain variable region sequences
  - Side effects (S.E.): infusion related, tumor lysis syndrome
- Alemtuzumab: monoclonal antibody against CD52, expressed on B and T cells
  - S.E.: immunosuppression
- Ibritumomab: murine antibody against CD20 with yttrium-90–labeled derivative
  - MOC: binds to CD20 on B-lymphocytes and delivers radioactive isotope, beta emitter.
  - S.E.: myelosuppression
- Tositumomab: murine anti-CD20 antibody conjugated to

iodine-131, gamma and beta emitter
- S.E.: infusion related, myelosuppression
- Gemtuzumab: humanized recombinant monoclonal antibody against CD33 linked to calicheamicin; an anticancer antibiotic
  - MOC: antibody to CD33 and delivers calicheamicin to immature normal and leukemic cells
  - S.E.: hepatotoxicity, myelosuppression

Estrogen Receptor Modulators

- Tamoxifen: nonselective estrogen receptor modular (ERM) that binds to estrogen receptors (ERs) in normal and malignant cells
  - Mechanism of action (MOA): binds to the ER and disrupts the estradiol–ER interaction
  - Estrogenic in the uterus, liver and bone; antiestrogenic in the breast
  - Side effects (S.E.): blood clots, endometrial cancer, hot flashes, vaginal discharge
- Aromatase inhibitors
  - Anastrazole, letrozole, exemestane.
  - MOA: inhibition of peripheral aromatization of androstenedione to estrone; blocks the conversion of androgens to estrone in peripheral tissues including fat, liver, muscle, and breast.
  - Anastrazole and letrozole are nonsteroidal competitive inhibitors.
  - Exemestane is a steroidal competitive aromatase inhibitor.
  - S.E.: Bone loss, hot flashes.
- Fulvestrant
  - Pure antiestrogen
  - MOA: competitive antagonist of ER, binds with affinity similar to estradiol, downregulates ER protein, has no ER agonist activity
  - S.E.: injection site pain, gastrointestinal

Antiandrogens

- Bicalutamide, flutamide, nilutamide
- Competitive antagonists on the interaction between androstenedione and the androgen receptor
- S.E.: gastrointestinal, feminizing side effects

Epidermal Growth Factor Receptor Antagonists

- Trastuzumab
  - HER-2/neu: a member of the epidermal growth factor receptor (EGFR).
  - Overexpression of HER-2/neu in breast is associated with a poor prognosis.
  - MOA: murine monoclonal antibody directed against overexpressed HER-2/neu protein.
  - S.E.: cardiac toxicity, especially when given concurrently with an anthracycline drug.
- Cetuximab
  - Humanized monoclonal antibody directed against EGFR
  - S.E.: asthenia, increased transaminases, skin toxicities
- Erlotinib and Iressa: binds to EGFRs; blocking downstream signals that order cells to reproduce.
  - Given orally.

Vascular Epidermal Growth Factor Inhibitors

- Bevacizumab: recombinant humanized anti-vascular epidermal growth factor (VEGF) monoclonal antibody
  - MOC: binds and neutralizes all forms of VEGF
  - S.E.: hypertension, thrombosis, bleeding

Targeted Drug to Tyrosine Kinase Domain of Activated Growth Factor

- Imatinib mesylate
  - Blocks the tyrosine kinase activity of several oncogenes; Bcr-Abl translocation, c-Kit (stem cell receptor), and platelet-derived growth factor receptor
  - S.E.: myelosuppression.

Hypercalcemia

- Hypercalcemia is one of the most common metabolic abnormalities in patients with cancer.
- Most common malignancies associated with hypercalcemia are squamous cell cancer of the lung, metastatic breast cancer, multiple myeloma, renal cancer, high-grade lymphoma, adult T-cell leukemia/lymphoma, and acute lymphocytic leukemia (ALL).

■ Pathophysiology

- Bone resorption by osteoclasts, parathyroid hormone–related peptide release

■ Clinical Manifestations

- General: weakness, malaise, weight loss, anorexia, pruritus, fatigue
- Central nervous system (CNS): mental status changes, confusion seizure, coma
- Cardiac: shortened QT interval on electrocardiogram (ECG), bradycardia, cardiac arrhythmias
- Gastrointestinal (GI): abdominal pain, nausea and vomiting, constipation
- Renal: polyuria, kidney stones, renal failure

■ Diagnosis

- 40% of plasma calcium is bound to albumin; only unbound calcium is physiologically active.
- Corrected total calcium: patient's calcium + [0.8 × (4.0 – patient's albumin)]
- Ionized calcium needs no correction.

■ Treatment

- Patients who are asymptomatic and calcium (Ca) level less than 12 mg/dL: observe, push fluids
- Patients who are symptomatic or Ca level is more than 12 mg/dL: aggressive hydration with normal saline, loop diuretics, bisphosphonates, steroids; treat underlying cancer

- Maintain urine output at 200 mL/hr
- Stop thiazide diuretics because can exacerbate hypercalcemia

Hyperviscosity

- Increase in whole blood viscosity, caused by increase in red blood cells (RBCs), white blood cells (WBCs), and most commonly immunoglobulins/paraproteins. Immunoglobulin M (IgM) is the most common paraprotein to cause hyperviscosity.
- Frequently observed in Waldenström macroglobulinemia, acute leukemia, or increased RBCs in polycythemia vera.

■ Clinical Manifestations

- Malaise, poor vision, headaches, neurologic symptoms, arterial clots, myocardial infarction, stroke, and vertigo

■ Treatment

- IgM hyperviscosity: plasmapheresis; plasma is removed and replaced with normal saline. Initiate chemotherapy for underlying process.
- Polycythemia vera: Treat with phlebotomy after diagnosis established.

Hyperleukocytosis

- Hyperleukocytosis is defined as a blood blast count of more than 100,000. The exact number at which to start aggressive treatment is controversial.
- Commonly seen in acute leukemia.

■ Pathophysiology

- Blast cells are larger and more "sticky" in the circulation, leading to stasis and mimicking a thrombosis.

■ Clinical Manifestations

- Leukostasis can occur anywhere, common in the lung, brain, or genitourinary (GU) tract.
- Pulmonary leukostasis: dyspnea, tachypnea, rales, respiratory failure.
- CNS leukostasis: headache, blurred vision, stroke symptoms with focal weakness.
- GU leukostasis: priapism, enlarged kidneys, hyperuricemia, renal failure.
- Pseudo-hyperkalemia, hypoglycemia, hypoxemia.

■ **Treatment**

- Leukapheresis if symptomatic or more than 100,000 leukocytes
- Hydroxyurea at high doses
- Allopurinol
- Alkalinize the urine with bicarbonate added to the intravenously (IV) administered fluids.
- Minimize RBC transfusion to prevent further increases in the viscosity.
- Start chemotherapy in prompt time frame.

Heparin Overdose

- The therapeutic goal of IV administered heparin is 1.5 to 2.5 times the normal control.
- The half-life is approximately 1 hour, making it an easy drug to manipulate.
- Low-molecular-weight heparins (LMWHs) are not monitored routinely and have a 4-hour half-life.
- Two conditions in which LMWHs should be monitored are extreme obesity and renal failure.

■ **Treatment**

- Patient with bleeding and on a continuous IV heparin drip: stop infusion, give protamine sulfate (1 mg of protamine sulfate neutralizes 100 units of heparin); must give slowly.
- Protamine sulfate neutralizes approximately 49% of LMWHs.

Warfarin Overdose

■ **Treatment**

The American College of Chest Physician guidelines are as follows:

- International normalized ratio (INR) more than therapeutic range but less than 5.0 and no significant bleeding: Lower the dose, omit the next dose, and resume therapy at a lower dose when the INR is in the therapeutic range. If the INR is only slightly above therapeutic range, dose reduction may not be necessary.
- INR more than 5.0 but less than 9.0, with no significant bleeding: Omit a dose or two, monitor the INR more frequently, and resume therapy at a lower dose when the INR is within therapeutic range. If the patient is a high risk for bleeding, omit two doses and give small amount of vitamin K (1–2 mg orally). More rapid reversal involves giving more vitamin K.

- INR more than 9.0, with no significant bleeding: Omit warfarin, give vitamin K 3–5 mg orally, closely monitor the INR, and if the INR is not substantially reduced in 24 to 48 hours, give additional vitamin K. Resume therapy at a lower dose.
- INR more than 20, with serious bleeding: Omit warfarin, give vitamin K 10 mg by slow IV infusion, supplement with fresh frozen plasma (FFP) or prothrombin complex concentrates.
- Life-threatening bleeding: Omit warfarin, give vitamin K 10 mg by slow IV infusion, start prothrombin complex concentrates. Repeat the process until bleeding stops.

Thrombotic Thrombocytopenic Purpura

- Thrombotic thrombocytopenic purpura (TTP) is a devastating disease without prompt recognition.

■ Pathophysiology

- Disorder of a deficiency of ADAMTS-13 activity, either congenital or acquired.
- ADAMTS-13 is a metalloprotease that cleaves the peptide bond of a mature von Willebrand factor (vWf).
- A deficient protease allows vWfs to become unusually large and sticky in the circulation.
- Under shear stress, the sticky factors bind platelets and form thrombi.
- RBCs are passively sheared when traversing blood vessels occluded by platelets and unusually large von Willebrand factor thrombi.

■ Diagnostic Criteria

- Only two diagnostic criteria are required for the diagnosis of TTP:
  1. Thrombocytopenia: usually very low (10 to 25 K)
  2. Microangiopathic hemolytic anemia (MAHA) visualized on peripheral blood smear; fragmented RBCs, helmet cells, schistocytes, and occasional nucleated RBCs
- Previously, the diagnosis of TTP was made by a pentad of features: thrombocytopenia, MAHA, fever, renal abnormalities, and neurologic symptoms.
- However, when and if the patient has all five, he or she will be seriously ill.
- Patients need to be diagnosed before developing all five symptoms of the pentad.
- Thus, the dyad (thrombocytopenia and MAHA) is sufficient criteria for a diagnosis of TTP.

■ Other Clinical Manifestations
- Neurologic symptoms: headache, confusion, coma
- Renal abnormalities: proteinuria, hematuria, renal failure more likely to be seen in hemolytic uremic syndrome
- Fever: nonspecific
- Abdominal pain: can be the presenting symptom of TTP
- Thrombotic and hemorrhagic complications
- Symptoms from low platelets rare; usually no purpura

Laboratory Findings
- Very low platelet count that drops dramatically fast.
- Platelet count can be spuriously high because of RBC fragmentation counted by automated particle counters.
- Leukocytosis can be seen.
- Lactate dehydrogenase (LDH) is almost always elevated into the thousand range.
- Elevated bilirubin; indirect bilirubin is the predominant component indicative of hemolysis.
- Normal coagulation profile.

■ Treatment
- Plasma exchange should be instituted immediately.
- Involves placing a large-bore vascular catheter for exchange.
- Patients should not receive platelet transfusions, unless absolutely required; platelets will add "fuel to the fire."
- Daily plasma exchange with FFP or cryo-supernatant, not cryoprecipitate (as this contains vWfs).
- Continue until platelet counts normalize and patient improves clinically.
- LDH normalizes by process of exchange; thus, it is not the best test to follow.
- Function of exchange: removal of vWf multimers and platelets and replacement of missing proteases.
- 90% of cases resolve with appropriate treatment.

Sickle Crisis

■ Acute Chest Syndrome
- Chest wall pain, pain with deep breath, fever, SOB.
- Clinically indistinguishable from pneumonia.
- Common cause of death in sickle cell disease.
- Findings: Chest x-ray can show infiltrates resembling an infection, PO_2 can be decreased and should be watched carefully.

■ Aplastic Crises

- Sudden decrease in marrow production most commonly from Parvovirus B19 infection.

■ Vaso-occlusive Crises

- Severe bone pain, joint pain, abdominal pain, all-over body pain.
- Occlusion of blood vessels by sickling cells.
- Infection, dehydration, and stress are precipitators.

■ Treatment

- Hospitalization.
- IV administered fluids.
- Oxygen supplementation, intubation if needed for acute chest syndrome (ACS).
- Empiric antibiotics.
- Analgesics, usually strong narcotics IV.
- Exchange blood transfusion (EBT), transfusing normal hemoglobin slowly in exchange for sickle cells, can be instituted.
- EBT indicated for stroke, priapism, ACS, multiorgan failure.
- Goal: to decrease hemoglobin S to less than 30%.

Venous Thromboembolism

- Venous thrombosis is the second leading cause of death in patients with cancer.
- Cancer is a thrombotic risk factor as exemplified by Trousseau syndrome (migratory thrombophlebitis in the setting of a solid tumor malignancy), which may be occult or predate the diagnosis.
- Cancer types most often correlated with thrombotic events are brain, ovarian, pancreatic, lung, and colon.
- Patients with cancer are undergoing surgery, chemotherapy, indwelling catheters, prolonged immobilization, hormonal therapy, and hypercoagulable states. All of these factors increase the thrombotic risk over the baseline malignant thrombotic risk.

■ Treatment

- LMWHs or warfarin.
- Some patients develop warfarin resistance and need to be placed on LMWHs continuously.

Massive Blood Transfusion

- Replacing the entire volume (5 liters) of a patient in less than 24 hours

- Usually in trauma patients
- Dilution or consumption of clotting factors, platelets, hemoglobin

■ **Laboratory Tests**

- Complete blood (cell) count (CBC), INR, activated partial thromboplastin time (aPTT), fibrinogen, D-dimers

■ **Treatment**

- Maintain a hematocrit of more than 30, platelet count more than 50,000, fibrinogen more than 150, and normal aPTT and INR.

Neutropenia/Sepsis

- Defined as an absolute neutrophil count (ANC) less than 1800/μL.
- Percentage of segmented and banded neutrophils multiplied by the total WBC count equals the ANC.
- Mild neutropenia is an ANC between 1000 and 1800/μL.
- Moderate neutropenia is an ANC between 500 and 1000/μL.
- Severe neutropenia is an ANC between 0 and 500/μL.
- Neutrophil levels are lower in some racial groups: Africans, African Americans, and Jewish individuals.
- Risks of infections are highest at 0 to 200/μL and the chronicity of the neutropenia.

■ **Clinical Manifestations**

- Throat/mouth infections, oral ulceration, pharyngitis, skin infections, sinopulmonary infections, septicemia, fever, mucosal abscesses

Diagnostic Evaluation

- If evidence of a fever (temperature > 100.5°F [38.1°C]), the patient should be pan-cultured. This is considered a medical emergency.

■ **Treatment**

- Institute aggressive evaluation and early institution of broad-spectrum antibiotics immediately.
- Avoid rectal or vaginal examination in a neutropenic patient because spontaneous bacteremia can occur with enteric/vaginal organisms.

Superior Vena Cava Syndrome

- External compression of the superior vena cava (SVC) by a tumor, usually lung cancer or lymphoma.

- Thrombosis of the SVC can be another nonmalignant cause in a patient with cancer.

■ Clinical Manifestations
- Facial edema, erythema, dyspnea, cough, and neck pain
- Hoarseness, dysphagia, lethargy, unable to lie flat

Diagnostic Evaluation
- Tissue biopsy is needed.

■ Treatment
- Chemotherapy or radiation should be given for underlying tumor.
- Diuretics and steroids can be given for symptom relief as workup proceeds.

Spinal Cord Compression

- Should be considered an emergency needing treatment immediately.
- Can result in irreversible paralysis, inability to walk, quadriplegia, and loss of bowel and bladder function.
- The most common tumors that cause cord compression are lung, breast, prostate, multiple myeloma, lymphoma, renal, and unknown primary.

■ Pathogenesis
- Extradural metastases impinging on the spinal canal

■ Clinical Manifestations
- Pain localized to the spine, radicular pain, paresthesias; pain is made worse by movement, coughing, lying down, sneezing, or straining of any kind.
- Next symptom is weakness.
- Urinary retention, constipation, and motor losses are advanced symptoms.

Diagnostic Evaluation
- Suspect in patients with cancer with back pain.
- Magnetic resonance imaging (MRI) scan is the best imaging study.

■ Treatment
- High-dose dexamethasone followed by daily dexamethasone
- Surgical consult from orthopedic specialist
- Radiation consult if a radiation-sensitive tumor

Brain Metastases

- More common than primary brain tumors
- Very poor prognostic sign; limited life expectancy with brain metastases
- Cancers that most commonly spread to brain: lung, breast, melanoma

■ Treatment

- Solitary and in a surgically operable area: surgical resection followed by radiation
- Steroids started as soon as possible to decrease surrounding edema

Hyperuricemia

- Hyperuricemia is mostly found in hematologic disorders such as leukemias, lymphomas, and myeloproliferative disorders.
- Rapidly proliferating tumors with rapid cell turnover are at the greatest risk for hyperuricemia.

■ Clinical Manifestations

- Gouty arthritis, renal dysfunction, and acute renal failure

Diagnostic Evaluation

- Elevated serum uric acid level, increased blood urea nitrogen and creatinine

■ Treatment

- Allopurinol, alkalinization of the urine, IV fluids, dialysis if impending renal failure

Tumor Lysis Syndrome

- Rapidly growing tumors have massive cell turnover, rapid release of cell contents into the bloodstream.
- Particularly common during chemotherapy treatment.
- Patients can develop renal failure and death if metabolic disturbances are not corrected.
- Commonly occurs in lymphomas.

■ Clinical Manifestations

- Hyperuricemia, hyperkalemia, hyperphosphatemia, hypocalcemia, renal failure

■ Prevention

- Alkalinization of the urine; allopurinol

■ Treatment

- Aggressive IV fluids; dialysis if needed

Index

Note: Page numbers followed by f refer to figures; those followed by t refer to tables; those followed by b refer to boxes.